SYNTEX CORPORATION

# Principles and Procedures for Evaluating the Toxicity of Household Substances

A Report Prepared by the

COMMITTEE FOR THE REVISION OF
NAS PUBLICATION 1138,
*Principles and Procedures for Evaluating the
Toxicity of Household Substances*

Under the Auspices of the

COMMITTEE ON TOXICOLOGY
Assembly of Life Sciences
National Research Council

NATIONAL ACADEMY OF SCIENCES

WASHINGTON, D.C.   1977

NOTICE: The project that is the subject of this report was approved by the Governing Board of the National Research Council, whose members are drawn from the Councils of the National Academy of Sciences, the National Academy of Engineering, and the Institute of Medicine. The members of the Committee responsible for the report were chosen for their special competences and with regard for appropriate balance.

This report has been reviewed by a group other than the authors according to procedures approved by a Report Review Committee consisting of members of the National Academy of Sciences, the National Academy of Engineering, and the Institute of Medicine.

Prepared under Contract No. CPSC-C-75-0018, U.S. Consumer Product Safety Commission, and Contract No. N00014-75-C-0718, Office of Naval Research, with the National Academy of Sciences, Advisory Center on Toxicology.

*Contract Monitors*
Dr. Robert M. Hehir, Consumer Product Safety Commission, Bethesda, Md. 20207
Dr. Robert K. Jennings, Office of Naval Research, Department of the Navy, Arlington, Va. 22217

Library of Congress Catalog Card Number 77-99199
International Standard Book Number 0-309-02644-X

*Available from:*
Printing and Publishing Office
National Academy of Sciences
2101 Constitution Avenue, N.W.
Washington, D.C. 20418

Printed in the United States of America

COMMITTEE TO REVISE NAS PUBLICATION 1138,
*Principles and Procedures for Evaluating the
Toxicity of Household Substances*

ROBERT G. TARDIFF, Environmental Protection Agency, *Chairman*
JOSEPH F. BORZELLECA, Medical College of Virginia, Virginia Commonwealth University
JOHN DOULL, University of Kansas Medical Center
EDWARD J. FAIRCHILD, National Institute for Occupational Safety and Health
W. GARY FLAMM, National Cancer Institute
RAYMOND D. HARBISON, Vanderbilt University School of Medicine
VICTOR G. LATIES, University of Rochester School of Medicine and Dentistry
MARSHALL STEINBERG, Department of the Army (presently with Tracor Jitco, Inc.)


*Subcommittee on Ingestion*

MARSHALL STEINBERG, Department of the Army, *Chairman*
GEORGE J. LEVINSKAS, Monsanto Company
FREDERICK SPERLING, Howard University


*Subcommittee on Chronic Toxicity*

JOHN DOULL, University of Kansas Medical Center, *Chairman*
MORENO L. KEPLINGER, Industrial Bio-Test Laboratories
TED A. LOOMIS, University of Washington School of Medicine
IAN C. MUNRO, Department of National Health and Welfare, Canada
NORBERT P. PAGE, National Institute for Occupational Safety and Health


*Subcommittee on Dermal and Eye Toxicity*

JOSEPH F. BORZELLECA, Medical College of Virginia, Virginia Commonwealth University, *Chairman*
JOHN F. GRIFFITH, The Procter and Gamble Company, *Vice-Chairman*
W. RICHARD GREEN, The Johns Hopkins Hospital
HOWARD I. MAIBACH, University of California School of Medicine

*Subcommittee on Inhalation Toxicity*

EDWARD J. FAIRCHILD, National Institute for Occupational Safety and Health, *Chairman*
WILLIAM M. BUSEY, Experimental Pathology Laboratories
J. WESLEY CLAYTON, JR., University of Arizona
J. DOUGLAS MacEWEN, University of California, Irvine
THEODORE R. TORKELSON, The Dow Chemical Company


*Subcommittee on Mutagenesis*

W. GARY FLAMM, National Cancer Institute, *Chairman*
DAVID J. BRUSICK, Litton Bionetics Research Laboratories
JOHN W. DRAKE, University of Illinois
SIDNEY GREEN, Food and Drug Administration


*Subcommittee on Reproduction and Teratogenesis*

RAYMOND D. HARBISON, Vanderbilt University School of Medicine, *Chairman*
KUNDAN S. KHERA, Department of National Health and Welfare, Canada
PAUL L. WRIGHT, Monsanto Company


*Subcommittee on Behavioral Toxicology*

VICTOR G. LATIES, University of Rochester School of Medicine and Dentistry, *Chairman*
PETER B. DEWS, Harvard Medical School
DONALD E. McMILLAN, University of North Carolina School of Medicine, Chapel Hill
STATA E. NORTON, University of Kansas Medical Center


*Staff Officer:* JACK A. WINSTEAD

# Contents

Principles and
Procedures for
Evaluating the
Toxicity of
Household
Substances

# *1* Introduction

In 1964 the Committee on Toxicology of the National Academy of Sciences-National Research Council published *Principles and Procedures for Evaluating the Toxicity of Household Substances* for use by the Food and Drug Administration in fulfilling its responsibilities under the Federal Hazardous Substances Act (FHSA). Primarily the document covered acute toxicity from ingestion, aspiration, percutaneous absorption, ocular and dermal contact, and inhalation. The Consumer Product Safety Commission has since been made responsible for the FHSA and other acts. Recognizing the substantial methodological advancements in toxicology and of expansion of concern from acute to chronic intoxication, the Commission in 1976 requested that the National Academy of Sciences review and amplify their earlier publication.

This report was prepared explicitly for use by the professional toxicologist engaged in either of two roles. It should assist the administrator in developing and recommending strategies for testing compounds and products (mixtures) for the purpose of rendering hazard/safety assessments for human exposure. To this end, the toxicologist will review critically and evaluate the adequacy, accuracy, and validity of the investigations and will coordinate and interpret the significance of the overall experimental toxicity profile. The report also should assist the toxicological investigator faced with the translation of guidelines into protocols and operational manuals for the various subspecialty areas of toxicology. Through the application of experience and professional

1

judgment, the experimentalist will implement the many-faceted aspects of dose-response studies, synthesize a unified and comprehensive approach, and define the resulting information to interpret its significance.

The report focuses on assessment of the toxicity of chemicals used in the household. However, the principles and procedures described herein are equally applicable to testing chemicals used outside the home, such as pesticides, industrial compounds, food additives, and environmental pollutants. The important aspect is the development of design strategies to address properly whatever problems are at issue. The potential routes of human exposure and intoxication, as well as the anticipated magnitude of exposure, must be accurately determined or closely approximated before a design strategy is selected. The experimental routes of administration are determined by the projected exposure routes of the product during use. Similarly, the degree of exposure (dose level and duration) that could be anticipated influences the selection of dosage levels and durations of exposure in the overall design of predictor studies. Chapters 2, 3, 4, and 5 describe the methodologies for administration of chemicals via various routes. Chapters 2 and 5 deal with the oral route, the former in acute (including aspiration) and subchronic studies and the latter in lifetime investigations. Chapter 3 focuses on dermal and ocular applications. Chapter 4 describes the complexities of inhalation exposures.

Selection of test protocols and experimental conditions is influenced also by physical and chemical characteristics of the product, such as solubility, vapor pressure, density, and reactivity. For instance, certain hydrocarbons are more likely to pose an aspiration hazard after ingestion; consequently, if such ingestion is suspected, there should be investigations to evaluate that possible hazard. When the structure of a compound under evaluation is similar to that of an agent whose toxicity has been characterized previously, investigators may suspect that their toxic properties and potency are also similar. Design modifications may then be aimed with greater specificity at more narrowly defined toxic end points.

When testing household products, the toxicologist is faced with evaluation of new agents whose toxicity is undefined. In most instances, the development of the toxicity profile is a stepwise process requiring continual judgmental intervention to insure the development of significant and interpretable data. Generally, the process requires the selection of the animal model(s), the execution of the various phases representing different degrees of exposure, and the evaluation of some specialized end points, such as reproductive anomalies.

Although economic and statistical considerations often dictate the selection of a rodent model such as the mouse or the rat, the model selected must give reasonable expectation of extrapolation to man. In the past, animal models have often accurately predicted human toxicoses from therapeutic agents and environmental materials; however, in previous strategies several species have been used to increase the probability of accurate prediction. In such circumstances, the toxicologist must decide empirically which sets of data are to be used in the final hazard analysis. Generally, such decisions have been made on the basis of the "most sensitive species tested."

An additional parameter in the selection of predictor species is species-specific or comparative metabolism (toxicokinetics and biotransformation). Frequently, organic compounds have been classed as "ultimate" or "proximal" toxicants (i.e., those directly responsible for toxic manifestations) and as "distant" toxins (i.e., those requiring transformation *in vivo* to a more active species). In both situations, enzymic mechanisms are also present within the organism to detoxify or inactivate the toxic molecules. The most extensive review of metabolic profiles—both activation and detoxication—has been compiled by Williams.[24]

There are many diverse metabolic pathways in mammalian organisms. Some pathways are species- and even strain-dependent, while others appear universal for the same compounds. Some pathways within a species are activated sequentially as the concentration of substrate is increased *in vivo*, a factor that impacts substantially on dosage selection, as well as on interpretation of data from different dose levels. For those chemicals requiring metabolic activation for toxic manifestations and for those requiring inactivation for detoxication, development of metabolic information on laboratory animals *in vivo* and in man, at least *in vitro*, should significantly affect the choice of more reliable animal models and may reduce the overall cost of the evaluation by decreasing the number of species. Equally important, such investigations generate data useful in the selection of exposure parameters by determining biological availability and half-life, predilection for target sites, and potency for accumulation, storage, and redistribution.

After selecting the animal models, the investigator can address the generation of the toxicity profile for the products to be tested. Toxicity profiles identify the organs and organ systems whose integrity, either genetic, biochemical or morphologic, has been compromised to the extent that normal functions are impaired or the organism's ability to respond to stimuli has been damaged. Structuring these studies with several logically spaced dosage levels is essential for several reasons: to confirm the observed effects by demonstrating increased intensity of physiological alterations with increasing dose levels; to describe lesions and their severity (reversibility vs. irreversibility); to generate data about the genesis of lesions from biochemical to histopathological and gross pathological; to demonstrate differential sensitivity of organs, thereby identifying the most sensitive target organ(s); to generate data on graduated effects, the slope of which can be analyzed to predict toxic effects at lower doses; and to produce data from which to estimate thresholds.

Because of the complexities of toxicological studies, an operational definition of "no observed effect" is necessary. Such a "no effect level" is impacted upon by differential sensitivity, varying species and strains, sensitivity and specificity of analytical methods in physiology and biochemistry, alternate metabolic profiles, etc.[12]

The core investigations by which toxicity is defined include acute, subchronic, and chronic toxicity tests as outlined in Chapters 2, 3, and 5. Prior to initiation of *in vivo* testing, some investigators conduct preliminary toxicity studies *in vitro*, using either mammalian or nonmammalian cells. *In vitro* toxicity testing can serve as a prescreen to compare inherent toxicity among compounds and mixtures by using relatively simple indices such as cell survival. Recently developed *in vitro* systems have been successfully used to assess mutagenic activity. Some investigators have concluded that demonstration of mutagenic activity in such assays is sufficient evidence for the carcinogenicity of a test agent, since several chemical carcinogens *in vivo* are also mutagens *in vitro*. Additional experimentation is required before *in vitro* assays can reliably replace *in vivo* tests of mutagenicity and oncogenicity in the hazard evaluation. On the other hand, these *in vitro* assays can be helpful in developing priorities among large numbers of compounds and products to be tested *in vivo* and in suggesting more specialized toxicity studies *in vivo*.

Acute toxicity studies are described in detail in Chapters 2, 3, and 4. Such studies can be an end in themselves when performed to assess hazard from single or multiple closely spaced doses. Often these investigations serve as range finders for the longer exposure studies by producing data concerning lethal levels and signs of intoxication. Reliable parameters such as the LD50 can be used to compare and determine relative acute hazards. The slope of the dose-response curve yields an index of the margin of safety.

The design of subchronic, or 90-day, studies is described in Chapter 2. Using a dose-response mode, multiple-exposure investigations are performed to identify pathologic lesions at the biochemical and histological levels with some measurements of the physiological status of critical organs. Signs of toxicity are carefully monitored during the exposure phase. All histopathologic lesions, with the exception of tumors, can usually be delineated in carefully designed and executed subchronic studies. The scope of experimentation can be expanded to include information on repair of damage by observing groups of subjects during a "recovery" phase. Data from the subchronic study are usually required for the planning and design of the chronic studies.

Lifetime, or chronic, studies, as described in Chapter 5, are highly complex but most useful in the definition of minimum-effect levels and essential in detecting the oncogenic properties of chemicals. Since the basic design of such tests prevents the discrimination between carcinogens acting by either the "one-stage" or "two-stage"[2,7,9] mechanisms, the evaluation of hazard from positive findings must of necessity be somewhat conservative until clarifying data are generated. A flexible design can produce data on the characteristics and severity of pathologic lesions, as well as on the rate of pathogenesis. A full spectrum of physiological and pathological changes and end points at the subcellular, cellular, organ, and whole-body levels can be assessed. The results from this sequence of experiments are translated by the toxicologist into a comprehensive profile of toxicity of the test agent.

Transmissable genetic damage is one of the more far-reaching toxic manifestations, as the adverse effects may be the legacy of future generations. Suspicion that a compound or product may be a mutagen can be obtained from structure-activity considerations, from data demonstrating localization of the agent in the gametes, or from observed activity within *in vitro* systems. The application of *in vitro* test systems, as compared to *in vivo* testing, is practical because of decreased cost and time. However, to assess hazard, *in vivo* assays such as the heritable translocation test are still required for confirmation of effects and for development of dose-response data that can be extrapolated to humans. The assay systems for detecting heritable genetic damage are described in Chapter 6, along with a logic for assessing mutagenic hazard by progression from simpler to more complex test systems.

Irreversible toxic manifestations of grave consequence are associated with adverse effects to the reproductive system and to the offspring. Reproductive anomalies range from sterility to derangements in the production of mother's milk. The adverse influences may occur at any time within the reproductive cycle of the organism. Toxic effects to the offspring range from mortality to morbidity as subtle as decreased body weight at birth. In perspective, weakening of the offspring in early life may lead to later physiological deficiencies. Pronounced reproductive anomalies are teratic or morphological defects observed in offspring at birth. These are usually related to a toxic intervention during organogenesis. Such morphological defects are often crippling. Of late, teratology has expanded to include not only morphological alterations but also biochemical, immunological, and behavioral deficits. However, the test procedures involved in these investigations are only in the experimental stages. Tests to assess reproductive toxicity, including birth defects, are described in Chapter 7. These tests are often the outgrowths of the subchronic toxicity studies.

Subchronic and chronic toxicity studies prescribe the observation of laboratory animals for signs of "unusual" behavior. At times, high doses of certain compounds can directly affect locomotor functions at peripheral sites.

However, the agents that directly affect the central nervous system (CNS) require definition and study to determine their relevance in the overall toxicity profile. Most important is the determination of whether the behavioral modifications occur at dose levels below those producing other functional organic damage.

Behavioral observations in the subchronic and chronic studies are relatively crude and nonquantitative. Consequently, subtle changes in behavior may go unnoticed. Chapter 8 describes and defines a research strategy and methodology for the study of agents suspected of having influence on the CNS to the extent that alterations in either general or operant behavior are manifest. The selection of compounds for these investigations, as well as other highly specific experiments, must be judicious to insure maximum use of resources with maximum return of information. When selecting compounds for detailed evaluation of behavioral effects, the following properties should be considered: lipid solubility, distribution to and residence time in the CNS, and observed gross effects in previous studies. Generally, behavioral studies, if used, will follow chronic investigations in the development of the toxicity profile for a given agent.

This document describes, in relatively abbreviated form, the state of the art in the various phases of toxicity testing. Because the inclusion of a complete treatise on all phases of toxicological assessments is virtually impossible and impractical, the reader is directed to several reference sources for additional information.

In the areas of basic precepts and concepts in toxicology, the texts of Casarett and Doull,[5] Loomis,[10] Boyd,[3] and DuBois and Geiling[6] should be consulted for comprehensive treatment of the subject. From these texts, insight can be gained into the concepts of dose-response, selection of animal models, conditions of experimentation, and interpretation and extrapolation of data. Paget[15] deals more specifically with development and application of methodology within various frameworks of safety evaluation. Disciplines within toxicology have also received comprehensive and independent treatment: the National Cancer Institute has promulgated guidelines[22] for carcinogenesis testing; the Canadian Health and Welfare[4] has developed a scholarly document dealing with carcinogenesis, mutagenesis, and teratogenesis; the proceedings[20] of a symposium jointly sponsored by the Society of Toxicology and the Association of Official Analytical Chemists addresses in detail safety evaluations and toxicity testing; Mello,[11] Weiss and Laties,[23] and Xintaras et al.[25] describe the complexities of behavioral toxicology; a report of the National Academy of Sciences[13] delineates approaches and techniques for the assessment of the inhalation toxicity of combustion products; Piotrowski[16] and Williams[24] develop the application of metabolic studies to toxicity testing; and Salsburg[17] displays insight into design and interpretation of chronic toxicity testing.

This report emphasizes household products and the evaluation of their safety. Other publications have dealt effectively with the safety evaluation of chemicals in other categories and for other uses: drugs,[1,26] cosmetics,[1] food additives,[1,14] environmental chemicals,[12] and pesticides.[21] All of these documents share in the fundamental concepts of toxicity testing despite modifications in design to address specific classes of agents and unique uses. Consequently, these references are useful resources.

The extrapolation of data from high to low doses and from laboratory animals to humans is the source of constant concern and attention and is in a state of dynamic development. Documents related to this subject have been cataloged into a bibliography by the Society of Toxicology.[19]

Some periodicals that address highly specialized areas of growth in toxicology and safety evaluations, and various journals that contain papers on the toxicity and development of test procedures, are listed in the Bibliography at the end of this chapter.

. Toxicity testing and safety evaluation have specific requirements for staff, facilities, and program. Staff, by virtue of their training and experience, must have demonstrated multidisciplinary expertise. The toxicologist should also be characterized by sound judgment, not only in design and conduct of these studies, but particularly in interpretation and application of findings to safety evaluation. A well-qualified support staff is essential to insure proper execution of experimentation.

Toxicity studies should be conducted in appropriately constructed and controlled facilities so that results and their interpretation are not compromised nor their reliability threatened. The accreditation of various components within the toxicology laboratory will assure the most effective environment and the highest-quality results. The American Association for the Accreditation of Laboratory Animal Care is highly regarded for its accreditation of animal facilities and programs of animal care. Clinical laboratories can also receive accreditation via either the Center for Disease Control or professional organizations. The facilities should be maintained in accordance with regulatory statutes such as the Animal Welfare Act and the Clinical Laboratory Improvement Act. In addition, the facilities should be designed, constructed, and maintained to insure minimum effect on the outside environment. Control of sewage effluents, air emissions, and solid waste[5] is essential to minimize the release of potentially hazardous and unaesthetic materials into the environment.

In toxicology programs, staff and facilities should be carefully selected so that the highest-quality studies and most reliable data can be produced. The most critical factors affecting toxicology programs are quality assurance, standard operating procedures, occupational safety and health, and accountability. In the near future, federal and professional guidelines will codify uniformity and minimum quality requirements for nonclinical laboratories.

The selection of laboratories on the basis of capabilities has been confusing at times. The *Toxicology Laboratory Survey*,[18] published by the Society of Toxicology, has cataloged the laboratories that engage in toxicity studies and listed their capabilities. The cost of various phases of the safety evaluation has been described by Gehring *et al.*[8]

The performance of toxicity tests with ample safety margins or relatively low risks does not assure absolute safety and does not negate the need for monitoring the health of exposed humans. There is a remote possibility that the biological models have erroneously predicted toxic potency. In addition, unanticipated high exposures resulting from accidents or abuse are a tangible threat and cause for concern. Consequently, prospective epidemiological surveillance of the target species, humans, is often essential with the introduction of a new chemical or product into the household.

## BIBLIOGRAPHY

Advances in Modern Toxicology. Washington, D.C., Hemisphere Publishing Corp.
Annual Review of Pharmacology and Toxicology. Palo Alto, Calif., Annual Reviews, Inc.
Cancer Research. Baltimore, Williams & Wilkins.
Critical Reviews in Toxicology. Cleveland, CRC Press.
Environmental Health Perspectives. Washington, D.C., Government Printing Office.
Journal of Toxicology and Environmental Health. Washington, D.C., Hemisphere Publishing Corp.
Mutation Research. Amsterdam, Elsevier Scientific Publishing Co.
Proceedings of the European Society of Toxicology. Amsterdam, Excerpta Medica Foundation; distributed in the United States by American Elsevier, New York. [Until 1974, Proceedings of the European Society for the Study of Drug Toxicity.]
Progress in Toxicology, Special Topics. New York, Springer-Verlag.
Teratology. Philadelphia, The Wistar Institute Press.
Toxicology. Limerick, Ireland, Elsevier/North Holland.
Toxicology and Applied Pharmacology. New York, Academic Press.
Veterinary Toxicology. Manhattan, Kansas, American College of Veterinary Toxicologists (Kansas State University).

## REFERENCES

1. Association of Food and Drug Officials of the United States. 1959. Appraisal of the Safety of Chemicals in Foods, Drugs and Cosmetics. Austin, Tex.
2. Berenblum, I., and P. Shubik. 1947. A new, quantitative, approach to the study of the stages of chemical carcinogenesis in the mouse's skin. Br. J. Cancer 1:383-391.
3. Boyd, E. M. 1972. Predictive Toxicometrics: Basic Methods for Estimating Poisonous Amounts of Foods, Drugs, and Other Agents. Bristol, Scientechnica Ltd.; distributed in the United States by Williams & Wilkins, Baltimore.
4. Canada, Health and Welfare Department. 1973. The Testing of Chemicals for Carcinogenicity, Mutagenicity and Teratogenicity. September.

5. Casarett, L. J., and J. Doull, eds. 1975. Toxicology: The Basic Science of Poisons. New York, Macmillan.
6. DuBois, K. P., and E. M. K. Geiling. 1959. Textbook of Toxicology. New York, Oxford University Press.
7. Friedewald, W. F., and P. Raus. 1944. The initiating and promoting elements in tumor production. An analysis of the effects of tar, benzpyrene, and methylcholanthrene on rabbit skin. J. Exp. Med. 80:101-126.
8. Gehring, P. J., V. K. Rowe, and S. B. McCollister. 1973. Toxicology: Cost/Time. Food Cosmet. Toxicol. 11:1097-1110.
9. Hueper, W. C., and W. D. Conway. 1964. Chemical Carcinogenesis and Cancers. Springfield, Ill., Charles C Thomas.
10. Loomis, T. A. 1974. Essentials of Toxicology, 2d ed. Philadelphia, Lea & Febiger.
11. Mello, N. K. 1975. Behavioral toxicology: A developing discipline. Fed. Proc. Fed. Am. Soc. Exp. Biol. 34:1832-1834.
12. National Academy of Sciences-National Research Council. 1975. Principles for Evaluating Chemicals in the Environment. Report prepared for the Environmental Protection Agency by the Environmental Studies Board and the Committee on Toxicology. Washington, D.C.
13. National Academy of Sciences-National Research Council, Committee on Toxicology. 1976. Fuels and Fuel Additives for Highway Vehicles and Their Combustion Products. A Guide to Evaluation of Their Potential Effects on Health. Washington, D.C.
14. National Academy of Sciences-National Research Council, Food Protection Committee. 1970. Evaluating the Safety of Food Chemicals. Washington, D.C.
15. Paget, G. E., ed. 1970. Methods in Toxicology. Oxford, Blackwell Scientific Publications.
16. Piotrowski, J. 1971. The Application of Metabolic and Excretion Kinetics to Problems of Industrial Toxicology. Prepared under the Special Foreign Currency Program of the National Library of Medicine. Washington, D.C., Government Printing Office.
17. Salsburg, D. S. In press. The statistical power of life-time studies in rodents to detect carcinogenicity in the presence of pharmacological activity. J. Toxicol. Environ. Health.
18. Society of Toxicology. 1976. Toxicology Laboratory Survey.
19. Society of Toxicology, Technical Committee. 1976. Extrapolation: Experimental Animals to Man and High to Low Doses; Bibliography.
20. Symposium on Safety Evaluation and Toxicological Tests and Procedures. 1975. J. Assoc. Off. Anal. Chem. 58:633-693.
21. U.S. Environmental Protection Agency. 1976. Data requirements to support reregistration of pesticide active ingredients and preliminary schedule of call-ins. Fed. Reg. 41:7218-7376.
22. U.S. National Cancer Institute, Division of Cancer Cause and Prevention. 1976. Guidelines for Carcinogen Bioassay in Small Rodents, by J. M. Sontag, N. P. Page, and U. Saffiotti. Washington, D.C., Government Printing Office. NCI Carcinogenesis Technical Report Series No. 1. DHEW Publication No. (NIH) 76-801.
23. Weiss, B., and V. G. Laties, eds. 1975. Behavioral Toxicology. New York, Plenum.
24. Williams, R. T. 1959. Detoxication Mechanisms: The Metabolism and Detoxication of Drugs, Toxic Substances and Other Organic Compounds. New York, John Wiley & Sons.
25. Xintaras, C., B. L. Johnson, and I. de Groot, eds. 1974. Behavioral Toxicology: Early Detection of Occupational Hazards. Washington, D.C., Government Printing Office. HEW Publication No. (NIOSH) 74-126.
26. Zbinden, G. 1963. Experimental and clinical aspects of drug toxicity. Adv. Pharmacol. 2:1-112.

# 2 Ingestion Exposure

## ACUTE INGESTION

The LD50 may be defined as the dose that is lethal to 50 percent of a group of treated animals. It is the most frequently determined index of toxicity. Federal legislation dealing with toxicity uses the acute LD50 as an index of toxicity, especially the acute oral LD50. Acute is defined either as a single dose or exposure, or fractions of a dose, when given over a short period. Oral dosage is administered by gavage. There are provisions for such determinations in a variety of federal regulations. Legislation enacted by the Congress has resulted in the Registry of Toxic Effects of Chemical Substances (formerly the Toxic Substances List). This document is directed specifically to the provision of guidelines that are responsive to the requirement of the Hazardous Substances Act. The most conspicuous value in the list is the LD50. The hazard data are incorporated into the labeling of packaging and even influence the type of package and the mode of transportation to be used when shipping a product.

The concept of the LD50, the median lethal dose, was developed by Trevan[27] as a graphic index of toxicity. He defined it as that unit dose per unit animal weight that would kill one-half of an "indefinitely large" group of animals using rigorously defined quantal data. Lower numerical values indicated greater toxicity than did higher ones. Only death and survival were noted; nonlethal effects, regardless of severity, were not considered. The intent was not to measure pharmacological effects. Trevan showed also that the same biological relations and mathematical principles applied to the evaluation of defined nonlethal pharmacological effects. When a sequence of doses was plotted against the corresponding percent response of groups receiving those dose levels, a sigmoid curve was obtained that was symmetrical if the dose progressions were logarithmic. The 50 percent or median point could readily be extrapolated and the standard deviation and slope calculated.

The slope shows the ratio between dose increment and response increment. Slopes from other experiments involving different compounds or animal species can be compared. A flat dose-mortality curve suggests a potential for cumulative toxicity and thus the need for a longer testing period. The steepness of the slope has been used to indicate safety when the potential dosage to be applied or the amount that might be accidentally ingested is considered. Within species or strains, divergent slopes of similarly acting substances indicate differences in mechanism or site of action. Parallel slopes may indicate similarity of action.

All commonly used graphic methods assume that the responses of the "indefinitely large" group will be normally distributed. Elaborate statistical methods for fitting the best line to values were developed by Bliss[3] and others. These methods became extremely useful in biological assays that required accurate comparison of one compound or sample with another. The graphic method also permits extrapolation to other dose-response levels.

Quantal data divide a test population into two groups, responders and nonresponders. It is necessary to define rigorously the test limits. Death or survival are more easily defined than are nonlethal responses in which gradations of response must be considered. The all-or-none principle, the quantal response, applies to each parameter being measured during an ED50, the median effective dose.

Pharmacological effects, including median values, should not be extrapolated to other species, strains, sexes, or animals whose state of health differs from test animals. Strictly speaking, any value obtained applies only to the species, strain, sex, age, and state of health of the animals under test.[8,16,29] However, the purpose of the measurement is to evaluate potential toxicity to humans. Therefore, one uses the values as an estimate of acute toxicity to humans. Wide variations of LD50 among mammalian species can have particular significance. They may indicate a problem in estimating potential toxicity in man. The median effective dose does not apply to a populace or the inhabitants of a region.

The LD50 has forensic value, and its estimation is necessary for compliance with legislation. It is important in characterizing industrial and accidental hazards that may have a fatal outcome. It may be calculated by any of a number of graphic and nongraphic methods. These numerical data can be calculated with data-processing equipment. Various microprocessors and a range of computers can facilitate data reduction and the generation of the desired calculations. The numerical values obtained by any of the diverse methods[26] and with limited numbers of animals conform closely to each other. Grading systems of toxicity, such as those of Gosselin *et al.*[14] or of Hodge and Sterner,[15] are based on such values, and slope is disregarded. Some methods,[10,26,28] using only a few animals per dose level, provide a good nongraphic estimate of the median dose, but do not provide a measurement of the slope of the dose-response curve. A large portion of toxicological data is expressed in terms of "range-finding" doses.

Many important factors that are the real determinants of acute toxicity are not evaluated by the LD50 and its slope. But many of these factors can be observed and evaluated during the course of an LD50 determination. Site and mechanism of action, early or delayed death, and recovery rate may be better indices of toxicity and, eventually, of hazard. Morbidity and/or pathogenesis may have more toxicological significance than mortality. Often the mortality potential is far less than the morbidity potential.[4,5,25] The LD50 also frequently serves as the basis for determining the doses to be used in subchronic and chronic studies.


## TEST PREPARATION

*Acute Oral LD50*    As previously indicated, there are two general methods of estimating an LD50: nongraphic methods, which do not assume normally distributed responses, and graphic methods, which do. The monographic method is exemplified by Thompson's Moving Average Method,[26] for which Weil[28] has developed tables for rapid and convenient calculation, including the standard deviation. Sigmoid curves or probit regressions exemplify the graphic method. All methods require that the test animals be randomly assigned to groups, that the log of the dose be used in the calculation, and that logarithmically separated progression of doses be used. Frequently, doses progress by 0.1 logs (multiples of 1.26) or 0.3 logs (multiples of 2), and four or more dose levels are used. Weil's tables for Thompson's Moving Average Method require four dose levels with equal logarithmic intervals between them and equal numbers of animals in each group. The tables permit the use of as few as 2 and as many as 10 animals per dose level. A numerical value for the LD50 can be obtained even when all animals survive at the two lower dose levels and all die at the two higher ones.

A commonly used graphic technique is the Litchfield-Wilcoxon Method of using probits.[19] The probits, in turn, can be converted to percent effect, derived from the relation of the area under the normal curve to the standard deviation.[3,11] Log dose and percent effect may be plotted directly, and a best-fitting regression line by inspection may be drawn. The LD50, LD16, and LD84 are read directly from the regression and fitted into an equation, then the slope is calculated. From nomograms one can extrapolate the homogeneity of the data and obtain factors for the calculation of the fiducial limits of the median dose and the slope. Neither dose intervals nor animal numbers are required to be equal. Four dose levels should be used. At least one should be more than the 50 percent effect level and one below. One level should be at either the 0 or 100 percent level.

The graphic and nongraphic methods each have advantages and disadvantages. The method of choice should be based on the information needed and the conditions of the test.

*Animal Data*    The test animals should be characterized as to species, strain, and physiological and morphological characteristics. There is no standardized animal that is suitable for all tests. Laboratories and breeders should collect and periodically review control data on their animals. It is extremely important that the test animals be randomly selected for the dose-level groups.

In acute studies, untreated controls are generally not necessary. The dose-response during the determination of an LD50 may be an internal control. If either unusual or oil vehicles or special dosing techniques are used, then two control groups—one receiving the vehicle and one with naive animals—should also be used. The vehicle controls should receive the largest volume of vehicle used when administering the test compound. Animals should be fasted before gavaging. Mice should be fasted for about 4 h, rats and rabbits overnight, and dogs for 24 h. LD50 values may differ by a factor of 2 when gavaged doses are administered to nonfasted animals.[4,5]

Hygiene and ambience are of prime importance. Appendix B contains details of laboratory animal care and maintenance. The impact of housing and animal care on test results cannot be overemphasized.

*Age, Weight, and Sex*    The responses of different age-groups are functions of organ maturation and regression, as well as enzyme activity development and scarcity. Dose responses differ according to the age and weight of the test animal.[18] Young rodents do not have their full complement of mixed-function hepatic-oxidative enzymes, but do have a complement of conjugating enzymes. The reverse is true for humans.[13] Older animals tend to obesity with consequent modifications of distribution and storage of chemicals. Older animals also have age-associated degeneration of the liver and kidney and both degeneration and regression of other organs and tissues. Patterns and rates of metabolism vary with age, strain, and species. They also vary with sex and among pregnant females. Estrus may modify female responses; pregnancy may cause drastic changes in responses. If females are to be used, they should be nulliparous and nonpregnant.

For LD50 determinations, rats weighing from 200 to 250 g and mice weighing from 20 to 30 g are often used. Pregnant animals should not be used because of the changes in sensitivity and biochemistry of the dams. Immature animals (21-35 days) may be used when attempting to estimate hazards to young humans who are often at greatest risk in regard to accidents involving household substances. However, these studies should be performed in addition to, rather than in lieu of, studies on mature animals. A variety of reasons prompt this approach, not the least of which is to permit comparison of effects with other compounds with as little variability as possible.

*Species and Strains of Animals*   Rats and mice of various strains are most commonly used for LD50 determinations. The principal advantage in using these animals is their relative uniformity and availability. In addition, many data have been accumulated on these species. However, the results obtained with them may not be uniformly reliable in predicting human responses and may show responses quite different from those of other species.

With some compounds, strain differences may be important. The differing responses of various species or strains to the acute effects of toxicants may be due to differences in absorption, distribution, excretion, and metabolism. With all species, the test animals should be acclimatized to the environment prior to dosing. Excessive coprophagy can be prevented by housing rodents in suspension cages instead of with bedding. The number of animals housed in individual cages should be uniform.[6] Crowding of animals alters the measured LD50. Ideally each animal should be individually caged, but this is often not possible within the resources available to test facilities.

*Preparation of Test Material*   Differences in the preparation of the test materials are probably responsible for many of the variations in LD50 values found in the literature for a given substance. This is in part due to the vehicles used to dissolve, suspend, or dilute the material. This is particularly true of oil-soluble materials. Preferably, liquid test materials should be given undiluted. When dilution is necessary, water is the diluent of choice if the test material is soluble and stable in water. Corn or cottonseed oils, which are used to dilute oil-soluble materials, may alter the absorption of the test substance. The oils may also cause catharsis. Solvents with known toxic properties should be avoided. With microsyringes, most liquids can be administered undiluted in sufficiently small volume to permit an accurate LD50 determination. Whenever possible the actual product should be tested.

It may be advisable to grind a solid in a ball mill or mortar before attempting to put it in solution or suspension. Where simple suspensions are not feasible, it may be necessary to use suspending agents such as carboxy-methylcellulose or guar gum. Oil-soluble solids are often encapsulated when dosing dogs, monkeys, and cats.

## TEST PROCEDURE

*Route of Administration*　The oral route is most commonly used in deter-minations of median lethal dose. The dose is administered via soft rubber or polyethylene tubing or a large ball-tip needle. The maximum volume of liquid that can be given depends on the animal's size. With rats this is usually in the neighborhood of 4 or 5 ml, although as much as 10 to 12 ml has been given. Great variability in concentration of test materials should be avoided. For materials that are insoluble in aqueous solution and that must be administered in oily vehicles, 1.5 to 2.0 ml is generally the upper limit because of the laxative effect. The determination of the LD50 of insoluble solids poses difficult practical problems because of the large amount of material that may have to be administered. The values may be difficult to interpret because they may be the result of graphic extrapolation rather than specific measurements. An adequate estimate of hazard is obtained for most purposes if animals survive single oral dosages of 5 or 10 g/kg.

*Observation Period*　The time at which deaths occur or signs appear or subside may be important, particularly if there is any tendency for deaths to be delayed. It is characteristic of such compounds as alkylating agents that death may occur as late as the second week of observation or, in some cases, later. A 14-day observation period is sufficient for most compounds. Animals demonstrating signs at the end of 14 days should be held until they either recover or die. Duration of observation should not be fixed; rather, it is de-termined by the toxic reactions, rate of onset, and length of recovery period. The return of food consumption and/or body weights to control levels are excellent indicators of recovery. When these are not achieved, the attainment of a plateau may be a signal to terminate the test.

*Recording of Signs*　Observations should be recorded systematically as they are made. Separate records should be maintained for each animal. They may reveal more than one mechanism at a given dose level.[4] Signs of intoxication may differ at different dosages. The onset and duration of signs of toxicity may suggest whether a pharmacologic action or organic damage has occurred. While checksheets are helpful for many of the standard types of symptoms, recorded observations must not be restricted to options provided in the checksheets. Physical examinations during acute toxicity tests should include, but are not limited to, observations of signs in skin and fur, eyes, and mucous membranes; genitourinary, gastrointestinal, respiratory, cardiovascular, and autonomic and central nervous systems; and somatomotor activities. Depending on clinical signs, investigators observing dogs and other large animals should use hematology and clinical chemistry tests for hepatotoxicity and nephrotoxicity. Particular attention should be directed to observations for the presence of tremors, convulsions, salivation, diarrhea, lethargy, sleep, coma, food consumption, and body weight changes, especially if survival exceeds 1 day. Time to death and rate of recovery are very important toxicity parameters. Delayed death may indicate significant potential for cumulative effects. These observations will provide useful information regarding the biochemical and pharmacological effects of the compound. Organ damage may be present without functional disturbances;[2] functional disturbances may be present without tissue injury that is detectable by standard histopathological techniques.[23]

*Weight Change of Animals*    A severe toxic effect may sometimes be discovered by comparing the weights of treated animals with controls. Surviving animals should be weighed at least once during as well as at the end of a 14-day period. A record of food and water intake should be maintained. Starvation influences pharmacological responses as well as the weight and water content of several organs.[24]

*Necropsies*    Necropsies of some of the surviving animals, as well as of those that die shortly after dosing, may provide valuable clues to the type of toxic effect produced by the test compound. Therefore, they should be a part of the general procedure. Gross pathological changes of the intestinal tract and of such organs as liver, kidneys, and spleen may be noted. If there is evidence of gross pathology, determination of the histopathology of the involved structures should be considered.

*Evaluation*    Ideally, to assess potential health hazards to humans, toxicity studies would be conducted only in those species of animals whose metabolism of the compound is similar to humans. Because comparative metabolism is unknown for many materials, and because studies in humans are rarely feasible, rodents make good initial test subjects. While extrapolation of the results to humans may not always be valid, the correlation is reasonably good for single oral doses. Materials highly toxic to rodents generally are highly toxic to humans. Relatively innocuous substances in one species are often quite harmless to the other. Relative sensitivity of various species is often more relevant for subchronic and chronic toxicity studies. Acute toxicity testing, if necessary, can be conducted in several species. A similar degree of toxicity in several species indicates that toxicity to humans probably would be comparable. Marked variation in the responses of different species calls for the assumption that man is at least as sensitive as the most sensitive species studied.

## SUBCHRONIC INGESTION

Subchronic studies are designed to determine the adverse effects of regularly repeated exposures over periods ranging from a few days to 6 months. Usually the study parameters are well defined. The exposure levels are normally lower than those found in acute studies. Death is usually not the end point, and the routes of exposure normally include the anticipated route of exposure for man. The intent is to define a level that produces "no observed effects" and a higher level that produces any adverse effect.

The evaluation procedures are generally more extensive and detailed than those used to support acute studies. These procedures may include neurological, behavioral, physiological, biochemical, hematological, and urine analyses, as well as food intake, body weight, and clinical observations. Postmortem studies, including gross and microscopic pathology, organ weights, and organ/body weight ratios are performed.

Quantitative measurements are made serially for most of these observations. All quantitative data should be examined by statistical comparison of treated and control animals. Definition of central tendency and test-population variability are analyzed whenever possible.

Studies may be conducted with either immature or mature animals. The human population at risk should guide selection. Care should be taken to determine if a higher dose acting on a specific site produces a different effect from that produced by a lower dose, as different dosages may affect different target organs and different target sites. Test materials may be given either by gavage or added to the diet or water. Acceptability to the animals of test diets should be considered when selecting the method of dosing. paired feeding studies may be required to demonstrate whether reduced food intake at high dose levels is a function of rejection of diet or toxic manifestation. Water consumption may be measured if indicated by test conditions.

If the test substance is to be added to the diet, the concentration may be expressed in parts of toxicant, by weight, per million parts of diet (ppm). Because the amount of food ingested in relation to body weight varies with age, a fixed concentration in the diet yields a decreasing dosage as the animal matures. When a more constant dosage is desired, the concentration of the toxicant in the food may be adjusted as the amount of food consumption changes so that a constant milligram per kilogram of body weight dosage is approximated. As the animals mature, the need for adjustment of the toxicant concentration in the diet disappears.

It is again preferable to select species whose metabolism of a toxicant is judged to be similar to that of humans. More specific information regarding the principles for the design of target-organ system studies is found in the National Academy of Sciences publication, *Principles for Evaluating Chemicals in the Environment*.[20]

The same production lot of a toxicant should be used for the entire sub-chronic study. If this is not possible, each batch of the test material must be chemically characterized. Qualitative and quantitative physicochemical methods (mass, infrared, or ultraviolet spectroscopy, etc.) may be used to monitor the contaminant and measure its stability. If the substance is administered in drinking water, water consumption must be measured.

Other factors, such as bioavailability, may influence test results and ultimate interpretation of data; however, it is not always practical to consider them.

Subacute studies require the use of a control group drawn from the same animal population as the test groups. Controls should be treated identically to test animals in all respects. Ideally, the only unique difference between test and control animals should be the presence or absence of the stresses produced by the test substance.

## EVALUATION OF THE ASPIRATION HAZARDS OF LIQUIDS

Aspiration is the inspiratory sucking into the lungs of a liquid or foreign body. An aspiration hazard exists when a substance can enter the lungs, whereas aspiration toxicity involves the type and extent of damage that is produced in the lungs. As in other toxicologic events, physical and/or pharmacologic effects may be observed. A physical effect may be characterized by local damage caused by irritants or corrosives and pharmacologic effects by systemic respiratory depressants.

The accidental aspiration of liquids from the mouth occurs in just a few seconds. During this brief time, the liquid flows from the back of the mouth through the glottis and into the respiratory tract. The volume of liquid aspirated is self-limiting in a conscious individual. As soon as the liquid enters the lung, normal physiological reflexes oppose further entry of liquid. These responses are a momentary reflex cessation of breathing and the more active, expulsive mechanism of coughing.

Some potentially hazardous liquids, commonly found in the home, can readily be aspirated if ingested. Liquids such as benzene, toluene, xylene, and petroleum distillates are listed as special hazards in the *Federal Hazardous Substances Act Regulations* [16 Code of Federal Regulations (CFR) 1500.14].[7] Aspiration of these liquids can produce chemical pneumonitis, pneumonia, and pulmonary edema. The *Regulations* require certain cautionary statements on the labels of those consumer products that contain 10 percent w/w of these substances [16 CFR 1500.14(b)(3)] and that have viscosities below 100 Saybolt Universal Seconds (SUS) at 38°C (100°F) [16 CFR 1500.83(a)(13)].

Many liquids have a low degree of toxicity when administered orally but are hazardous if aspirated. For kerosene, the ratio of the oral LD50 to the intratracheal LD50 is 140 to 1 in the rat. This gives some idea of the relative magnitude of toxicity by these routes.[12] The volume of a single swallow in a child in the age-group at highest risk (1 to 5 yr) is approximately 1 teaspoonful.[17] Arena[1] suggested that aspiration of as little as 0.5 teaspoonful (2.5 ml) of kerosene could produce death in a young child. The aspiration of 1 ml of kerosene directly into the lungs of a child can produce severe chemical pneumonitis.[9]

The percentage of a mouthful of liquid that is aspirated either during drinking or emesis has not been determined. Rat data have shown that the amount of a petroleum distillate that can be aspirated is inversely proportional to its viscosity.

The viscosity of a liquid determines the probability of its being aspirated. Animal experiments have shown that aspirated petroleum distillates, and products that contain them, having viscosities below 100 SUS at 38°C produce the greatest increases in lung weight and mortality. These substances generally produce aspiration LD50's of approximately 1 ml/kg. Because distillates and products containing petroleum distillates have higher viscosities, they produce less lung edema and mortality in 24 h, while exhibiting aspiration LD50's of 2 to 3 ml/kg.[22]

Using radiolabeled petroleum distillates, investigators have demonstrated in rats that approximately 70 percent of an oral dose (1 ml/kg) is aspirated when a petroleum distillate with a viscosity of 30 SUS at 38°C is administered. When the viscosity is increased to 363 SUS at 38°C, approximately 40 percent of the same dose is aspirated.

Volume is also a determinant. About 70 percent of a 1 ml/kg dose (30 SUS at 38°C) can be aspirated in contrast to approximately 3 percent of a 0.1 ml/kg dose of the same oil.[21,22] This clearly indicates that the amount of liquid that enters the lung is determined by the dose and its viscosity.

Rat data have also confirmed the aspiration hazards of high-viscosity oils (above 100 SUS at 38°C). Investigators have observed a delayed (14 days postaspiration) inflammatory, lipoid pneumonia response in the lungs.[22]

Surface tension (which is the measure of the spreading tendency of a liquid) might also be expected to influence the pulmonary distribution of an aspirated liquid. Surface tension of petroleum distillates varies only slightly in contrast to their wide range of viscosities. Therefore, surface tension is not an important factor in the range of aspiration toxicity of various petroleum distillates. However, it may significant for aspirable substances other than petroleum distillates.

## TEST PROCEDURE

Approximately 25 percent of a petroleum distillate dose (1 mg/kg) enters the lungs when it is instilled in the trachea as compared to 70 percent when applied by the method described by Gerarde[12] and modified by Osterberg et al.[21] The modified method relies on the production of increased lung weight and/or lung/body weight ratio, higher mortality ratio, and altered physical appearance of the lungs. A combination of these factors is used as a basis for predicting potential aspiration hazard. The dose volumes used reflect accidental ingestion levels of children, based on a 10-kg child.

Although test methods described below focus on petroleum distillates, they are also applicable to other liquids.

In the modified method albino rats of either sex, weighing from 200 to 300 g, are used. The rats are anesthetized with ethyl ether to the point of slow diaphragmatic breathing, which may be rapidly followed by apnea. The anesthetized rat is placed in a supine position at an approximate 120° angle to the table top, with its head elevated. Its mouth is held open by a hemostat inserted between the jaws. The tongue is pulled forward and held with forceps. This prevents the swallowing reflex. Doses of 0.25, 0.5, or 1.0 ml/kg are delivered into the rear portion of the mouth near the tracheal orifice. The nostrils are held closed by the investigator's fingers, thereby forcing the rat to breathe through its mouth. The rat is maintained in that position until either the characteristic sounds of one or two aspirations (slurps) are heard and the investigator judges that the test material has entered the trachea or the rat shows signs of regaining consciousness. The nostrils and tongue are then released, and the rat is returned to a holding cage. If the investigator believes that the rat has not aspirated the dose, that animal is eliminated from the test.

Control groups of rats receive distilled water in place of an oil. Following aspiration all rats are observed for 24 h and given free access to food and water. The lungs of those rats that die are immediately removed and weighted. Animals showing signs of rigor mortis are not used due to postmortem changes. Twenty-four-hour survivors are exsanguinated following ether anesthesia. Their lungs are also quickly removed. Only lungs that show no external signs of overt murine pneumonia or of trauma are used.

The lungs are gently blotted on disposable tissues or gauze sponges. Lung weights are obtained to the nearest centigram (0.01 g). Analyses of lung weight and lung/body weight ratios and mortality data can be compared with the control group using standard statistical tests. Surgical excision techniques must be standardized to avoid surgically induced variations in lung/body weight ratios.

## EVALUATION

Products are considered to be hazardous if they produce either statistically significant increases in lung/body weight ratios with visible lung congestion in surviving rats, more than a 25 percent increase in lung weight, or a statistically significant mortality ratio in the test group.

## REFERENCES

1. Arena, J. M. 1973. Poisoning, 3d ed. Springfield, Ill., Charles C Thomas. p. 198.
2. Balazs, T., and H. C. Grice. 1963. The relationship between liver necrosis and pentobarbital sleeping time in rats. Toxicol. Appl. Pharmacol. 5:387-391.
3. Bliss, C. I. 1938. The determination of the dosage-mortality curve from small numbers. Q. J. Pharm. Pharmacol. 11:192-216.
4. Boyd, E. M. 1959. The acute oral toxicity of acetylsalicylic acid. Toxicol. Appl. Pharmacol. 1:229-239.
5. Boyd, E. M., M. Dolman, L. M. Knight, and P. E. Sheppard. 1965. The chronic oral toxicity of caffeine. Can. J. Physiol. Pharmacol. 43:995-1007.
6. Casarett, L. J., and J. Doull, eds. 1975. Toxicology: The Basic Science of Poisons. New York, Macmillan.
7. Consumer Product Safety Commission. 1976. Products requiring special labeling under section 3(b) of the act. 16 CFR 1500.14.
8. Cram, R. L., M. R. Juchau, and J. R. Fouts. 1965. Differences in hepatic drug metabolism in various rabbit strains before and after pretreatment with phenobarbital. Proc. Soc. Exp. Biol. Med. 118:872-875.
9. Deichmann, W. B., and H. W. Gerarde. 1964. Symptomatology and Therapy of Toxicological Emergencies. New York, Academic Press. p. 236.
10. Deichmann, W. B., and E. G. Mergard. 1948. Comparative evaluation of methods employed to express the degree of toxicity of a compound. J. Ind. Hyg. Toxicol. 30:373-378.
11. Finney, D. J. 1971. Probit Analysis, 3d ed. Cambridge, The University Press.
12. Gerarde, H. W. 1963. Toxicological studies on hydrocarbons. IX. The aspiration hazard and toxicity of hydrocarbons and hydrocarbon mixtures. Arch. Environ. Health 6:329-341.
13. Gillette, J. R., and B. Stripp. 1975. Pre- and postnatal enzyme capacity for drug metabolite production. Fed. Proc. Fed. Am. Soc. Exp. Biol. 34:172-178.
14. Gosselin, R. E., H. C. Hodge, R. P. Smith, and M. N. Gleason. 1976. Clinical Toxicology of Commercial Products—Acute Poisoning, 4th ed. Baltimore, Williams & Wilkins.
15. Hodge, H. C., and J. H. Sterner. 1949. Tabulation of toxicity classes. Am. Ind. Hyg. Assoc. Q. 10:93-96.

16. Hurst, E. W. 1958. Sexual differences in the toxicity and therapeutic action of chemical substances. *In:* Walpole, A. L., and A. Spinks, eds. The Evaluation of Drug Toxicity. London, J. & A. Churchill, Ltd. pp. 12-25.
17. Jones, D. V., and C. E. Work. 1961. Volume of a swallow. Am. J. Dis. Child. 102:427.
18. Lamanna, C., and E. R. Hart. 1968. Relationship of lethal toxic dose to body weight of the mouse. Toxicol. Appl. Pharmacol. 13:307-315.
19. Litchfield, J. T., Jr., and F. Wilcoxon. 1949. A simplified method of evaluating dose-effect experiments. J. Pharmacol. Exp. Ther. 96:99-113.
20. National Academy of Sciences-National Research Council. 1975. Principles for Evaluating Chemicals in the Environment. Report prepared for the Environmental Protection Agency by the Environmental Studies Board and the Committee on Toxicology. Washington, D.C.
21. Osterberg, R. E., S. P. Bayard, and A. G. Ulsamer. 1976. Appraisal of existing methodology in aspiration toxicity testing. J. Assoc. Off. Anal. Chem. 59:516-525.
22. Osterberg, R. E., R. Johnson, G. Bierbower, and J. McLaughlin, Jr. 1975. An evaluation of petroleum distillates as aspiration hazards in rats. Toxicol. Appl. Pharmacol. 33:195. Abstract no. 185.
23. Paget, G. E., ed. 1970. Methods in Toxicology. Oxford, Blackwell Scientific Publications.
24. Peters, J. M., and E. M. Boyd. 1965. Organ weights and water levels in albino rats following fortnight starvation. Toxicol. Appl. Pharmacol. 7:494-495. Abstract no. 52.
25. Smyth, H. F., Jr., C. P. Carpenter, and C. S. Weil. 1951. Range-finding toxicity data: List IV. AMA Arch. Ind. Hyg. Occup. Med. 4:119-122.
26. Thompson, W. R. 1947. Use of moving averages and interpolation to estimate median effective dose. I. Fundamental formulas, estimation of error, and relation to other methods. Bacteriol. Rev. 11:115-145.
27. Trevan, J. W. 1927. The error of determination of toxicity. Proc. R. Soc. London Ser. B 101:483-514.
28. Weil, C. S. 1952. Tables for convenient calculation of median-effective dose (LD50 or ED50) and instructions in their use. Biometrics 8:249-263.
29. Weil, C. S., C. P. Carpenter, J. S. West, and H. F. Smyth, Jr. 1966. Reproducibility of single oral dose toxicity testing. Am. Ind. Hyg. Assoc. J. 27:483-487.

# 3 Dermal and Eye Toxicity Tests

This chapter is concerned with several types of tests commonly used to assess acute hazards of chemicals to skin and eyes. In addition, types of hazards for which there are presently no standard tests are included in order to address a perceived need for such tests.

For several years much attention has been given to improving the reproducibility and reliability of some of these tests through standardization of technique and interpretation. Relatively little attention has been directed to the toxicological principles upon which the tests are based. Therefore, this chapter places more emphasis on these principles. Doing so has led to some suggestions for departures from or alternatives to present, familiar procedures that have recognized deficiencies. The fundamental guideline has been that, to predict hazard to humans, a test result must be gauged against standards for which human response or experience is known.

Whether or not a new test is needed or changes in an existing test are in order, standardization of any procedure should involve extensive interlaboratory validation and a program for uniform training of persons who will perform and interpret it.

## ACUTE DERMAL TOXICITY

A test for acute dermal toxicity should evaluate the potential for systemic toxic effects of chemicals expected to come in contact with the skin. In practice this is done by determining the median lethal dose (LD50) of a single dermal exposure to the animal species under test. As that LD50 is used in hazard evaluation of household substances, the test conditions should be related to anticipated human exposure.

Dermal toxicity is one of the three categories of toxicity defined by route of exposure in the Federal Hazardous Substances Act (FHSA). This act further defines a "highly toxic" substance in this category as one that "produces death within fourteen days in half or more than half of a group of ten or more rabbits tested in a dosage of two hundred milligrams or less per kilogram of body weight, when administered by continuous contact with the bare skin for twenty-four hours or less" [16 CFR 1500.3(b)(6)(i)(C); see Appendix A]. An alternative definition for "highly toxic" and one for "toxic" by the dermal route appear in more conventional toxicological terms in the FHSA *Regulations* [1500.3(c)(1)(ii)(C) and (2)(iii)]. A description of a test method that specifies the use of rabbits appears in the same document (1500.40; see Appendix A). These statutory definitions place constraints on the conduct of acute dermal toxicity tests performed in accordance with present regulations. Nevertheless, in the following discussion, attention will be given, where appropriate, to principles and procedures that are desirable alternatives to those presently specified.

## TEST PREPARATION

The dermal toxicity test in rabbits specified in the FHSA *Regulations* is described by Draize et al.[18] They suggest using, in addition to rabbits, such animal species as the mouse, rat, guinea pig, or dog. The monkey, cat, goat, and swine have also been used.[40] The adult albino rabbit has been the preferred species for such reasons as size, ease of handling, and restraint, and because its skin is the most permeable of all species studied. However, the rabbit appears to be almost exquisitely sensitive to dermal insult, and elicited reactions may not be valid for humans. The skin of swine and the guinea pig have permeability characteristics more like those of humans. The albino rat is somewhat less reactive than the rabbit and more reactive than the guinea pig or humans. The rat should be a preferred species because it is the one most used for LD50 studies by other routes of exposure and for other types of toxicological studies.[21,52] Also, there are more sources supplying high-quality, disease-free rats than of like quality rabbits in the United States.

The following weight ranges are suggested: male rats, 200 to 300 g; female rats, 180 to 250 g; rabbits (male or female), 2.3 to 3.5 kg (cf. 1500.3 and 1500.40 for specific requirements); male guinea pigs, 350 to 450 g; and female guinea pigs, 400 to 425 g. Shortly before testing, fur from the trunk of healthy, previously unused animals should be clipped so that no less than 10 percent of the body surface area is available for application of material. Care should be taken to avoid abrading the skin, which could alter its permeability. The present FHSA *Regulations* calls for making epidermal abrasions every 2 or 3 cm longitudinally over the area of exposure on "approximately one-half of the animals." In testing of household products it would be more appropriate to conduct tests on normal, intact skin. Reasons for this are given in the section on skin irritancy testing. However, if a dermal LD50 for abraded skin is desired, the skin of test animals should be abraded.

## TEST PROCEDURE

The material to be evaluated should usually be tested in its commercial form unless this form is unlikely to come in contact with the human skin. With solids, it may be desirable to moisten the skin and the test material with saline. Finely divided solids can be applied uniformly to gauze, which is then placed against the skin. For some applications it may be appropriate or necessary to use a vehicle. If such is the case, any effect of the vehicle on the penetration of the test compound should be established.[40]

The maximum quantity of a liquid test substance to be applied is 2 ml/kg; for a solid or semisolid test substance, the maximum is 2 g/kg of body weight. The dose should be applied uniformly over not less than 10 percent of the body surface area, but not more than 30 percent. At least three doses should be tested to permit adequate assessment of dose-response relationships. Animals should be restrained during application of the material.

The test dose must remain in contact with the skin throughout the exposure period. In some procedures, e.g., for liquids, this is done by applying the dose inside an impermeable cuff made of rubber dam or plastic film. Such devices occlude the skin, thereby enhancing penetration and potential toxicity of the test material. For this reason routine use of occlusive dressings is not recommended unless anticipated human exposure warrants it. Liquid or solid doses can be held in contact with the skin with a porous gauze dressing.

A 4-h exposure is recommended unless continuous skin contact is anticipated in humans. Weil *et al.*[66] found that the rat 4-h dermal LD50's and the rabbit 24-h dermal LD50's tend to rank materials in the same order.

During a 4-h exposure, animals can be prevented from ingesting the test material by immobilizing them. During exposures as long as 24-h, immobilization of rabbits or guinea pigs may impose undesirable stress. Restrainers that permit animals to move about their cages, plus some form of screen or other device to cover the applied material, may be useful in such cases. Rats, having far greater agility, require more restraint than rabbits. When animals are tested with volatile substances having appreciable toxicity, it is also important to prevent inhalation exposure.[20]

The number of animals per dosage group depends on the level of statistical confidence desired. Ten animals per dose is recommended in most cases. For materials of anticipated low toxicity, an initial range-finding dose of 2 g/kg of body weight applied to five or more animals may be sufficient to demonstrate a lack of appreciable dermal toxicity.

At the end of the exposure period, any residual material is gently removed with a gauze compress, the exposed area examined, and any lesions noted (see section below on skin irritation). Animals are then returned to their individual cages with *ad libitum* access to feed and water. For 14 days the animals should be examined at least daily for signs of systemic toxicity and localized dermal reactions.

The method of calculating the acute dermal LD50 is the same as that described in Chapter 2 for the acute oral LD50 for animals.

All animals that succumb or are moribund are necropsied. At the end of the 14-day observation period, all survivors are subjected to a thorough examination, including examination of the exposed area of skin. They are then sacrificed and necropsied. The degree of skin irritation, signs of intoxication, changes in body weight, mortality, and gross pathological findings as a function of dose and time are noted.

## EVALUATION

The acute dermal LD50, as well as the acute oral LD50, are convenient for estimating toxic hazard. Although there is always risk in extrapolation from animals to humans, it is usually safe to presume that substances with lower dermal LD50's in animals will be potentially more toxic to humans than those with higher LD50's. On the other hand, predictions of dermal versus oral toxicity in humans are more difficult, especially if the dermal and oral measurements are made in different animal species. Therefore, there is an important advantage in having both tests done with the same species, e.g., the rat.

## PERCUTANEOUS PENETRATION

Percutaneous penetration refers to the transfer of a chemical from the skin's surface into the body, including entering the epidermis and the dermis, and systemic absorption. Various methods measure different aspects. The kinetics of percutaneous penetration comprise at least 10 steps, not all of which can readily be quantitated.[44] The extent of a chemical's penetration of human skin must be determined to ensure prudent extrapolations from acute and chronic toxicological data that have been generated in animal assays.

The two animals whose percutaneous penetration is closest to humans are the monkey and the domestic swine.[2,44,68,69] Unfortunately, correlation data are available for only a few compounds. Data exist for only one anatomical site—the forearm. Animals can be reused when the chemical is no longer detectable.

Percutaneous penetration is dose-related; however, it is not necessarily linear and depends on the compound and the vehicle. The dose should be determined in relation to probable human exposure. Most published experimental human data are for doses of 4 $\mu g/cm^2$. If practical, the anatomical site dosed should be relevant to the eventual human exposure. The number of animals must be determined on the basis of the information that will be required. The variation in percutaneous penetration is large. In groups of three to six animals, a standard deviation of 30 percent can be expected.

Vehicle selection is important. Volatile solvents such as acetone have been widely used because they evaporate rapidly, leaving the test chemical in place. Most percutaneous penetration studies are single exposures. It is convenient to express application quantities in micrograms/square centimeter. Multiple dosing may not necessarily produce more penetration than one dose. One or more standard compounds should be included in the test series to facilitate comparison with the known animal and human toxicological data.

Most percutaneous penetration studies performed in animals quantitate a chemical or a radioactive tracer appearing in the urine, feces, bile, and sometimes in the expired air. The skin may hold chemicals for long periods; therefore, collection of biological fluid will usually last for a minimum of 5 days. The method of quantitation may be chemical, a radioactivity measurement, a radioimmunoassay, or other. It is customary to express the amount of absorption in terms of the dose applied. It is mandatory to ascertain whether the chemical would in fact be excreted and not stored in the body. A parenteral control is obtained, usually by intravenous dosing of a similar tracer dose of the chemical chosen in relationship to the amount that might penetrate. If 50 percent of the dose was accounted for in the urine on the basis of the intravenous control, the penetration from the skin would be assumed to be at least twice that measured in the urine.

Considerable information is available from human testing, which can usually be performed rapidly and safely once the appropriate animal toxicology has been completed. There is some correlation between *in vitro* data obtained with human skin and *in vivo* data from human testing,[13,62] but the relationship must be better understood before *in vitro* tests can be used for routine screening of chemicals.

## SKIN IRRITATION

A reliable test for skin irritation should provide a means for differentiating among substances that will produce different degrees of irritation or corrosion of the skin. In this context, irritation is the local inflammatory response of normal living skin to direct injury by single, repeated, or prolonged contact with a chemical agent without the involvement of an immunologic mechanism. The macroscopic manifestations are erythema and edema. Corrosion is direct chemical action on normal living skin that results in its disintegration and irreversible alteration at the site of contact. Its important manifestations are ulceration, necrosis, and, with time, the formation of scar tissue. It is especially important to be able to distinguish between materials that will produce minor or inconsequential degrees of skin irritation from materials that can produce substantial irritant or corrosive injury as a result of customary or accidental exposure.

The voluminous literature on primary irritation test methods lacks consensus on the animal model or procedure most likely to give accurate and dependable results. Test procedures for human subjects are as numerous as those for animals, suggesting that the problem does not lie solely in selection of the test species. The most standardized animal procedure is that of Draize et al.[18] as it is adopted for household products in 16 CFR 1500.41 (see Appendix A). This is a 24-h, semiocclusive patch test of a full-strength product on both intact and abraded skin of albino rabbits. A modification with exposure time shortened to 4 h and the detailed evaluation of corrosive effects has been proposed.[65] This proposal, with the requirement for testing abraded skin deleted, has been adopted by the Department of Transportation for identifying corrosive substances (49 CFR 173.240; see Appendix A).

The effects on skin of various forms of products concern manufacturers, consumers, and regulatory bodies. They should be considered in any safety assessment of household substances. There may be skin irritation hazards during the use of products in undiluted, diluted, or mixed form. Discussion here, however, must be limited to the testing of undiluted materials as they are obtained in their original packages. It is not feasible to discuss in proper balance the testing of all customary forms of products to which one might be exposed. Furthermore, the discussion will be limited to tests involving single exposure with the recognition that they will not reveal cumulative effects that could result from recurrent exposures under realistic conditions of use. If cumulative effects are of concern, they can be evaluated by other techniques.[15,19,34,38,42,47,61]

## TEST PREPARATION: ANIMAL TESTING

Most of the conventional laboratory animals and some of the more exotic species and domestic breeds have been tried in skin irritancy testing. None provide perfect models for human skin. The albino guinea pig and albino rabbit, though commonly used, lack the human repertoire of responses to skin irritants. They show only degrees of erythema and edema. Both species, but especially the rabbit, react more strongly than humans to mild-to-moderate irritants. In fact, some materials that appear unsafe when tested on rabbits may be nonirritating to human skin.[51,61] The response of guinea pig skin is more like that of human skin over a wide range of materials. In addition, the guinea pig's requirement for space and caging is more economical. For these reasons the guinea pig is preferable to the rabbit.[25,56] Young adult guinea pigs of the albino Hartley strain are suitable. The New Zealand white is most often specified if a test on rabbits is desired.

## TEST PROCEDURE: ANIMAL TESTING

The usual procedure is to place 0.5 g of the test substance on the skin under a gauze pad or other inert, semiabsorbent material. Liquids and semisolids can be applied directly, but solids, powders, and the like should be moistened with solvent. A 50 percent slurry or solution is convenient. Various sizes of patch have been prescribed,[17,55] ranging from less than 1 to 4 in.$^2$ This determines the dose per unit area of skin that affects the amount of response. As most existing data have been obtained using the Draize procedure, 0.5 g on a 1-in.$^2$ pad (i.e., 0.5 g/in.$^2$), the same size patch is desirable for inter-laboratory comparability. Several patch materials can be used effectively, including 2-ply or 12-ply gauze, nonwoven cotton fabric, or cellulose pads. The material selected should be inert to the test material. It should also be capable of containing a liquid or moist material without completely absorbing it and thereby reducing contact with the skin.

To prepare animals, the fur should be clipped from their backs, taking care not to scrape the skin. Two patches can be applied to a guinea pig, one to either side of the midline of the back. Four patches can be placed on a rabbit. The patches are held in place with narrow strips of adhesive tape. A porous type of tape is preferred to minimize occlusion.

After the desired number of patches is applied, the animal should be loosely wrapped with a semiocclusive covering such as rubberized cloth or stockinette. This secures the patches and prevents their removal by the animal. The placement of collars on animals may also prevent them from removing the patches. For a short application period, an alternative is to restrain the animals.

Each material should be applied to test sites on six separate animals. By using two sites on each guinea pig, it is possible to test two materials on each animal.

In any group of materials to be tested, it is desirable to include a comparison standard of known human skin irritancy. The composition and properties of this material should be similar to the test substance, if possible. The most useful controls are those that can be compared to human response.

The Draize procedure and that described in 16 CFR 1500.41 (see Appendix A) call for an equal number of skin sites to be abraded before application of the test material. This may be appropriate for testing drugs and cosmetics intended for use on diseased or damaged skin, but it provides no relevant information on other types of products. The skin of laboratory animals is usually more reactive than human skin. Abraded skin imposes an additional degree of exaggeration that is difficult to interpret. In addition, abrasion techniques are difficult to standardize. Nixon et al.[51] have shown that classifications of irritancy based only on intact skin are not usually different from those using abraded skin. Therefore, the use of abraded skin is not recommended.

It has been recommended that the 24-h patch test of Draize be shortened to 4 h when testing household substances[65] and materials transported interstate (49 CFR 173.240; see Appendix A). Exposures to household substances are usually of short duration. This modification precludes exaggerated exposure of animal skin that is more reactive than human skin. The Committee recommends a 4-h application of the patch test. However, there may be types of products for which either longer or shorter patch tests would approximate use exposures more realistically. For example, it might be satisfactory to use a shorter application time for materials that will evaporate and be less likely to remain on the skin. Nonvolatile residues from compositions that are predominantly volatile may be tested by first allowing a few minutes for evaporation before applying or covering the patch. At the end of the 4-h period, the patches should be removed and the skin site gently cleansed with water. To remove some substances, it may be necessary to use a nonirritating solvent other than water. If there is any doubt about irritancy, control sites should be tested with empty or water-moistened patches and then cleaned with the desired solvent to establish a baseline response. For materials that are very difficult or impossible to remove from the skin, it may be necessary to read peripheral areas or take skin sections for histological examination.

## EVALUATION: ANIMAL TESTING

After removal of the test materials, 30 to 60 min should lapse before the patch sites are read to allow sufficient time for pressure and hydration effects to subside. Additional readings should be made 24 and 72 h after the patch application. On the other hand, persistent effects such as corrosion are better determined at 7 days. In some cases, it may be useful to retain animals for 2 wk after application. Because such delayed readings usually only confirm effects seen at 7 days, their value should be measured against the cost of maintaining the animals.

Responses after 4, 24, and 72 h are conveniently scored by using the dual, erythema-edema scale of Draize *et al.*[18]

*Erythema and Eschar Formation*

| | |
|---|---|
| No erythema | 0 |
| Very slight erythema (barely perceptible) | 1 |
| Well-defined erythema | 2 |
| Moderate to severe erythema | 3 |
| Severe erythema (beet redness) to slight eschar formation (injuries in depth) | 4 |
| Total possible erythema score | 4 |

*Edema Formation*

| | |
|---|---|
| No edema | 0 |
| Very slight edema (barely perceptible) | 1 |
| Slight edema (edges of area well defined by definite raising) | 2 |
| Moderate edema (raised approximately 1 mm) | 3 |
| Severe edema (raised more than 1 mm and extending beyond area of exposure) | 4 |
| Total possible edema score | 4 |

It is customary to add the erythema and edema scores at each grading, though this gives equal weight to the separate parameters and may not be entirely appropriate for some types of reactions. Different types of materials may produce maximum irritant responses at different times. As the practice of averaging scores taken at various times (e.g., 4, 24, and 72 h) tends to obscure peak responses, it would be better to base the irritancy evaluation on only the highest mean score for the test group at either 4, 24, or 72 h.

Persistent or delayed effects, such as those seen at 7 or 14 days, should not be graded by the irritation scale used for acute responses; they should be evaluated for presence and extent of ulceration necrosis or scarring.

It is tempting to assign categories of irritancy to ranges of scores or irritation indices, as this would seem to simplify predictive evaluations. Unfortunately, absolute scores are subject to considerable inter- and intralaboratory variation.[67] Though such variation might be reduced by more standardized training in test techniques, the evaluation of test scores relative to comparison standards with which there is human experience is a more reliable approach. The irritation score obtained with the test substance is compared with that of a known nonirritant or irritant with similar chemical and physical properties and rated accordingly. Comparison standards may also be used in predicting degrees of corrosiveness.

## TEST PREPARATION: HUMAN TESTING

When appropriate, e.g., following a screening test in animals and with proper attention to ethics, tests on human volunteers are preferred to animal tests if it is important to avoid the uncertainties of interspecies extrapolation. Human subjects should be of consenting age and may be of either sex. It has not been shown that one race is more responsive to irritants than another, though slight inflammatory reactions are more easily detected on light skin.[33] Tests for skin irritancy with human subjects may be performed if responses are generally limited to superficial inflammatory effects and do not injure the subject. Materials of unknown or unfamiliar composition should be tested first on animal skin to establish the conditions under which they can safely be applied to humans. If a substance could be a strong sensitizer or be uniquely damaging to human skin, trial exposures of short duration or with diluted material should be made. These precautions should ensure testing of substances without causing severe responses. Before any test involving experimental exposures of humans, fully informed consent of the subjects should be obtained.

## TEST PROCEDURE: HUMAN TESTING

It is desirable to use more human than animal subjects in patch testing because of the greater range of individual variability among human volunteers. Ten subjects is a satisfactory number in an acute test.

The FHSA defines an irritant by the response it produces on normal living tissue. Therefore, the use of abraded skin is not recommended. Also, pigmentary changes within abrasions will sometimes leave undesirable marks on the skin.

The procedure is similar to that used with animals. Patches may be applied to the intrascapular area of the back or to the dorsal surface of the upper arms. Because 8 to 10 patches can be applied to each subject, 1 or more patches for comparison standards can be applied simultaneously. In place of the wrapping around the bodies of animals, a large piece of porous adhesive tape can be used to hold patches on human subjects. Care should be taken to vary systematically the order that patches are placed on a test group of subjects, because some patch locations receive more pressure than others and have better contact. This pressure could be caused by clothing, leaning against chair backs, and so forth. Skin reactivity can also differ from one region of the body to another.

A single exposure of 4 h is suggested, though it may be necessary (and sufficient) to use shorter exposures with strong irritants or very volatile materials. Subjects should be instructed to remove patches immediately if they cause pain or unusual discomfort. During continued exposure, pain may diminish while damage is increasing. In such a case the patch site should be examined as soon as possible after the patch is removed.

At the end of the exposure period, patches should be removed and the skin cleansed with water or a nonirritating solvent to remove residual material.


## EVALUATION: HUMAN TESTING

The responses at each patch site should be evaluated 30 min to 1 h after removal of the patch to allow time for pressure and hydration effects to subside and again 24 h after the patch was removed. Each patch site should also be examined 3 to 4 days after application to determine if any delayed or persistent reactions are present.

There are many scales for scoring human skin responses. Some of them rate separately such visible responses as redness and swelling. Other scales integrate redness and swelling and may also include such phenomena as papule formation and vesiculation. The points on any scale are arbitrary. The adding of separate scale points or averaging scores involves quantitative assumptions about data that are primarily judgmental. Nevertheless, it is a common and convenient practice to calculate means or indexes from scores obtained in this way.

The dual Draize scales for redness and swelling can be used for grading human skin responses. They are easy to learn, but have no provision for scoring papular, vesicular, or bullous reactions or reactions that spread beyond the site of application. For this reason, many investigators prefer an integrated scale such as the following one, which is based on the scale of Marzulli and Maibach:[47]

| | | |
|---|---|---|
| 0 | = | no response |
| 1/2 or + | = | questionable or faint, indistinct erythema |
| 1 | = | well-defined erythema |
| 2 | = | erythema with slight-to-moderate edema |
| 3 | = | vesicles (small blisters) or papules (small circumscribed elevations) |
| 4 | = | bullous (large blister), spreading, or other severe reaction |

Scores assigned from this scale may be averaged for all subjects and compared with the average score produced by standards of known irritancy. If the average score for the test material differs markedly from that for the standard (e.g., 1.0), it is advisable to retest it against another standard. This will permit a more precise prediction of its potential irritancy.

## PHOTOTOXICITY

A phototoxic response refers to irritation (not immunologically mediated) that depends on light exposure for its presence. This does not refer to irritation occurring without ultraviolet light, nor to that which is only aggravated by light. The latter is a secondary response and is an additive irritant effect. The purpose of testing is to determine whether a chemical has phototoxic potential. The phototoxic chemical studied most extensively is bergapten (5-methoxypsoralen), for which the hairless mouse, the rabbit, and humans have similar, particularly strong reactions. The guinea pig and swine show less response; the squirrel, monkey, and hamster are refractory to bergapten.

### TEST PROCEDURE

Animals are exposed by applying the chemical in a solvent. It is important to be aware of the possibility that solvents may react with the chemical or otherwise absorb energy on exposure to ultraviolet light, thereby altering the test situation significantly. Dosing should be on a microgram- or milligram-per-square-centimeter basis, simplifying the extrapolation to dosing in humans. The skin site can be conveniently demarcated with a marking pen. The chemical can be delivered to the skin with a micropipette. Following application, the animals are exposed to ultraviolet light from a high-output source. Most responses to phototoxic chemicals are elicited by high-intensity, ultraviolet light above 310 nm. This simplifies testing, as it is possible to filter out shorter, erythema-producing wavelengths. For compounds that elicit responses below 310 nm, a different testing system is mandated.[46]

It is customary to administer one high dose. No situation has yet been found in which a compound has been negative at a high dose and positive at a low dose. If the high dose is positive, the least effective dose is then determined. Each animal may be used as his own control. Controls include negative (the vehicle), positive (a known relevant phototoxic chemical such as bergapten), and unirradiated, chemical-treated sites. Experience suggests that most chemicals that are phototoxic by cutaneous exposure will produce toxicity in most animals if given in a sufficient dose. Small groups, from 4 to 10 animals, are sufficient for this testing.

The phototoxic response is usually elicited quickly. For maximum effect the site should be irradiated within 30 min to 2 h after the chemical application. Grading is performed 12 to 24 h later. The parameter most generally measured is a visible and palpable dermatitis, consisting of erythema, induration, and at times frank necrosis. The Draize system is the reference scale presently available. The combination scales, including erythema and edema, are convenient alternates. Both systems are fully described in the section on irritation. The phototoxic response is dramatic; there are few easier tests to read. Certain chemicals and solvents irritate the skin. When this occurs, attempts should be made to decrease the effective tissue dose so that the irritancy is not seen in the site not exposed to light. Standard statistical tests for significance may be used to evaluate the resulting data.

Occasionally, extrapolation to humans of results obtained from animal phototoxicity tests may be questionable. In such cases, tests with humans may be necessary if the basic systemic toxicologic data are available. The experimental procedure resembles that used with animals; however, because human skin is less permeable than that of most small laboratory animals, it is usually necessary to make the skin more permeable by removing most of the stratum corneum with repeated cellophane tape stripping. A stripped skin site control is also used. The dose should be administered in one small application.

## CHANGES IN PIGMENTATION

Pigmentation may either decrease (hypopigmentation) or increase (hyperpigmentation). The greatest concern is depigmentation. Many, if not most, cases of chemically induced leukoderma mimic vitiligo and are often misdiagnosed as such. It may be necessary to determine the proclivity of some household substances to produce depigmentation in humans. The greatest amount of experimental data has been obtained with the pigmented guinea pig. There is reasonable correlation of effectiveness between those chemicals known to produce depigmentation in the guinea pig and those producing it in humans. Methods for testing chemicals for their tendency to produce depigmentation have been published.[8,22,45]

## CHLORACNE

Chloracne may result from exposure to any of several industrial chlorocarbons. The eruption produced may be severe and last for months to years; therefore, it is important to identify those household substances containing chlorohydrocarbons that may produce chloracne in humans. The clinical features are most consistent, helping to establish the syndrome as a unique form of acne. The adult albino rabbit, which has been systematically studied, develops chloracne from exposure to those chemicals known to produce chloracne in man. Methods to evaluate chemicals' proclivity to produce chloracne have deen described.[1,28,29,59]

## DELAYED-TYPE CONTACT SENSITIZATION

Delayed-type allergic contact sensitization refers to an immunologically mediated cutaneous reaction to a chemical. With few exceptions, contact sensitization develops as a result of one or more contacts with a chemical that initiates the sensitization process. The latent sensitized condition generally develops no sooner than 1 to 2 wk after the effective exposure. Subsequent exposure of the skin of the sensitized individual to a sufficient concentration of the sensitizer or related substance (cross-sensitizer) can elicit a more intense response than previously. This response may take hours or even days to develop, hence it is "delayed." Responses may be characterized by pruritis, erythema, edema or induration, papules, vesicles, bullae, or combinations of these. Reactions generally subside over a period of days if there is no further contact with the sensitizer, but the state of sensitization may be permanent.

A test should demonstrate a strong potential for sensitization by a chemical or product. It should detect materials that are capable of inducing either a substantial incidence or degree of sensitization responses among individuals exposed during use or accidental misuse.

### TEST PREPARATION: ANIMAL TESTING

Laboratory animal species are generally much less responsive to contact sensitizers than humans. The guinea pig is the most responsive, particularly the albino varieties. The strain of guinea pig selected should be readily capable of sensitization by a (common) allergen such as chlorodinitrobenzene. Animals from 1 to 3 mo of age are preferred, as they are more sensitizable than very young or older animals. There is no appreciable difference in the proclivity of male and female guinea pigs to develop sensitization, but pregnant females should be avoided. Animals are generally not reused; however, sensitized animals may be useful in tests for cross-sensitizers or other sources of a given sensitizer.

Animals should be quarantined for a minimum of 1 wk to ensure that they are free of infection. Hair should be removed from their backs, sides, and flanks by clipping, shaving, or depilation.

### TEST PROCEDURE: ANIMAL TESTING

The guinea pig standard tests are derived from observations of Landsteiner and Jacobs.[37] The most generally used technique is that of Draize et al.[18] In one version, approximately 10 healthy young adult albino guinea pigs are selected. An area of skin between the shoulder blades is exposed first by clipping and then shaving. A 0.1 percent solution or suspension of the test material in saline is injected intradermally into the shaved skin. Injections of 0.1 ml are repeated thrice weekly for a total of nine, keeping the injections within a 3 to 4 cm$^2$ field. Two weeks later the animals are challenged with 0.05 ml of the test solution injected into a fresh site. The animal is considered sensitized if the challenge reaction is noticeably greater than the reactions to the inducing injections.

In some cases, it is preferable to give an equivalent amount in four intradermal injections at one time, using a dose several times greater than that producing minimal perceptible irritation. This dose is determined in a preliminary dose range-finding study. If after one challenge (performed as above) the animals are not sensitized, the intradermal injections and challenge are repeated—in essence a doubled-up Draize procedure.

In practice, all variants of the Draize procedure require that the final challenge be of minimal or no irritancy in the control animals. As irritation produces a heightened (nonimmunologic) responsiveness, it is important not to misinterpret such false positive reactions. To help avoid this, one can use an unrelated nonsensitizing chemical of similar irritancy to the test chemical as a negative control. Even with the use of controls, intradermal injection procedures can produce localized irritation reactions at injection sites that may be misinterpreted by inexperienced investigators as sensitization.

An alternate technique takes advantage of the ability of guinea pig skin to tolerate rather high concentrations of topically applied chemicals without excessive irritation. Groups of 15 to 20 animals are patch-tested with the substance for 6 to 24 h once weekly for 3 wk. The patches must have an occlusive backing to enhance penetration of the test substance. Following a rest period of 1 or 2 wk the animals are rechallenged with a high, but nonmarginally irritating concentration of the test solution and the vehicle on separate sites. Using the topical route, substances may be detected that are not demarcated by the intradermal method.[10]

Another means of enhancing the sensitivity of the guinea pig is by using Freund's adjuvant, either mixed with the putative allergen or injected separately (split-adjuvant techniques).[43]

Extensive data document the value of combining topical, intradermal, and Freund's adjuvant exposures.[31] A row of three injections is made on each side of the midline. These injections are:

- 0.1 ml of adjuvant (without the test agent)
- 0.1 ml of test agent without the adjuvant
- 0.1 ml of test agent (approximately 5 percent) emulsified in complete adjuvant

One week later the topical application is made after pretreatment for 24 h with 10 percent sodium lauryl sulfate in petrolatum, which enhances penetration and sensitization by provoking a mild inflammatory reaction. Challenge is made with a 25 percent concentration or the highest subirritating concentration.

When sensitization testing is performed with a dilution of the material, it is best to employ a vehicle permitting solubilization. The vehicle should allow release of the chemical and should not react with it. Common vehicles include water, ethanol, acetone, propylene glycol, vegetable oils, petrolatum, and various preparations of surfactants and emulsifiers. Experience usually indicates the one type of vehicle that is more convenient to use with a given class of compound.

The quantity of test material is usually expressed as a given volume (usually standardized for a given technique) and concentration. The concentration should exceed that projected for human exposure. Although excessively high doses could induce tolerance rather than sensitization, there is a greater risk of failing to detect a sensitizer by using too low a concentration. Within practical limits, there is a greater likelihood of obtaining sensitization by increasing the number of doses (intradermal or topical).[17]

## EVALUATION: ANIMAL TESTING

Because cutaneous responses are visible, they can be readily evaluated by a trained observer. An arbitrary scale of 0 to 4+ or any other system may be used, provided that the investigator accurately describes what is seen. Basically, the degree of erythema and the amount of induration or edema palpated should be recorded. Vesiculation and necrosis, which may also occur, should be noted accordingly.

The delayed reactions of contact sensitization are best evaluated by making sequential observations of test sites on the skin. The first should be made 24 h after injection or removal of a patch to allow primary irritation to subside. A second reading should be made 24 or 48 h later.

Reactions to the test substance at challenge that are stronger than reactions to negative controls or to those seen during induction should be suspected as results of sensitization. Responses that are marginally more intense than control response or that occur in very few animals should be confirmed by a second challenge after 1 or 2 wk. Rechallenge after a longer delay can be unreliable, as sensitization in guinea pigs is short-lived compared to that in humans. Whether or not a rechallenge is performed, a judgment confirming the presence or absence of sensitization should be made and recorded for each animal. Mean scores or indices, which are customarily calculated for each experimental group, are useful only for showing relative intensity of response.

Two or more unequivocally positive responses in a group of 10 to 20 animals should be considered significant. A negative, equivocal, or single response probably assures that a substance is not a strong sensitizer, though this is best confirmed by further testing with human subjects.

## TEST PREPARATION: HUMAN TESTING

There has been considerable experience with human sensitization assays, most of which were derived from the animal assays described above. In the majority of these, the test substance is applied topically under an occlusive bandage. Occlusion of the skin greatly enhances penetration and makes the test more sensitive.

## TEST PROCEDURE: HUMAN TESTING

There are basic procedures with useful variations. The first is the repeated insult technique of Draize[17] and Shelanski and Shelanski.[58] The test material (usually 0.5 g or 0.5 ml) is applied under occlusive patches to the dorsal skin of the upper arm or the interscapular area of the back in repeated doses for a total of 9 to 15 applications. The concentration used should exceed the exposure anticipated during use unless this would produce excessive irritation. The patches are applied on alternate days and removed after 24 h. Some investigators prefer a 48-h application. It is usually feasible to test four or more materials simultaneously, though in so doing one must be aware of the possibility of cross-reactivity between similar materials. After this initial series of induction patches, no more patches are applied for 10 to 20 days to allow time for latent sensitization to develop. Subjects are then challenged with the test material for 24 to 48 h. Responses are evaluated 3 and 5 days after the patches are applied.

The second procedure is the maximization test,[32] which is based on the premise that most chemicals have some sensitization potential for humans. This can best be determined if the epidermal barrier to percutaneous penetration is breached. This is usually accomplished by substantially irritating the skin with sodium lauryl sulfate before and one or two times during the series of applications of the test substance. Five sequential patches are applied to volar surface of the forearm, each for 48 h with 24 h between. There is then a 10-day waiting period, followed by further irritation of the skin with sodium lauryl sulfate, after which a challenge patch is applied.

More subjects are needed than in guinea pig tests because of greater range of immunologic responsiveness among humans and the lower concentrations of materials that may be required. Draize[17] originally specified that 200 subjects should be used. This is reasonable in seeking weak sensitizers in cosmetics and topical drugs, but is probably not necessary for detecting moderate-to-strong sensitizers encountered in exposures to other types of household products. Prudence dictates that materials showing possible weak sensitization in guinea pigs should be tested on only a few human volunteers at a time. If no human response is found, the numerical base can be expanded. The maximization procedure has been standardized at 25 subjects; 50 to 100 subjects are commonly tested in the repeated insult test.

## EVALUATION: HUMAN TESTING

Human skin manifests a greater variety of visible responses (e.g., erythema, edema, induration, papules, vesicles, bullae) than guinea pig skin. Consequently, grading scales are more complex. Any scale that can be adequately described can be used. All reactions should be noted during the induction phase of the test and at two intervals after the challenge, e.g., 2 and 4 days.

Sensitization should be distinguished from primary irritation, as both may occur simultaneously. The length of a reaction is important to note. Irritant responses often begin to disappear within a day or two once the contactant is removed. Sensitization responses, which may develop more slowly and persist longer, tend to be characterized by induration, papules, or vesiculation. Any suspected sensitization response should be confirmed by a rechallenge test 2 wk to 2 mo after the initial challenge and after earlier reactions have subsided. Although this type of testing appears deceptively simple, both experience and judgment are required to perform it adequately.[48] The inexperienced investigator would benefit by working with an experienced investigator before initiating trials.

## CONTACT URTICARIA

Skin responses to chemical contactants, if immunologically mediated, are usually delayed-type hypersensitivity. However, the wheal and flare of urticaria can occur directly from skin contact with some chemicals. This is important not only in terms of the local response: With percutaneous absorption, the response may become generalized. In more sensitive individuals or after large antigen exposure, angioedema, asthma, and anaphylactoid reactions can occur. Nonimmunological contact urticarial reactions may also occur.

The limited testing for contact urticariogenicity suggests that experienced investigators should be able to detect it during conventional tests for delayed-type contact hypersensitivity. When a urticarial response is suspected, special techniques can be employed to determine whether it is immunological or nonimmunological and whether the substance has an important potential for producing the effect. The immediate sensitivity test is performed on intact or scratched skin using a control such as citraconic anhydride.[27] The guinea pig is an animal of choice; human testing has been performed.[53]

## EYE IRRITATION

Test procedures to assess the surface toxicity of liquids, solids, and aerosols to ocular tissues of laboratory animals should show the potential for substantial human eye injury. There are several reported procedures, but that of Draize *et al.*[18] is the basis not only of the method specified in the FHSA *Regulations* (16 CFR 1500.42; see Appendix A), but also of several other accepted methods. The evaluation of gases in eye irritation requires special techniques, as exposures may be sustained. The Draize rabbit eye irritation test[18] has been widely criticized for its poor reproducibility and its inaccurate reflection or prediction of human experience.[11] Yet there is no practical test generally available that is less empirical or more reliable. Therefore, in the following discussion, emphasis will be placed on ways to improve the Draize test by means that are feasible for most modern toxicology laboratories.

### TEST PREPARATION

*Selection of Animal Model* Historically, eyes from albino rabbits have been used in most test procedures, apparently because they are large and have no pigmentation. In addition, the tractable nature of the animal facilitates handling and examination. However, the rabbit eye differs in several anatomical and physiological respects from the human eye. The structure of the cornea is thinner, the nictitating membrane is well developed (third eyelid), the fur surrounding the eye and on the lids is thick, the blink reflex is not well developed, and irritation causes tearing.

Limited comparative data from controlled exposures of humans and rabbits show responses of the rabbit eye to be much more severe and long-lasting injury.[4] Other nonprimate laboratory species such as rats, guinea pigs, dogs, and cats are either less satisfactory than rabbits or have not been thoroughly evaluated. Among nonhuman primates, rhesus monkeys have been used the most,[5,12,23] but cynomolgus and squirrel monkeys are also suitable. The potential use of monkey species as human models seems obvious; their eyes are structurally and functionally similar to humans. Unfortunately, the limited availability, cost, and hazards in the handling of monkeys prevent their extensive use. Therefore, the albino rabbit is the species of choice, with the monkey (especially the rhesus) as the preferred second species when confirmatory data are necessary.

Ocular responses of rabbits are not known to be sex- or age-dependent, but healthy, sexually mature animals of either sex less than 2 yr old are recommended. Albino rabbits are preferred to pigmented strains to facilitate observing iris changes. When using monkeys, sexually immature animals are preferred.

In a given test, only one eye of each animal should be used, and the animal should not be subjected to extraneous test procedures or stresses. The contralateral eye may be used for another test after the first eye has returned to normal.

Eyes to be tested should be free of defects or injury and should not stain with fluorescein. This can be best determined by gross examination on the day before the start of a test. Animals should be housed in clean cages that are free of particulate bedding material or other extraneous substances that could irritate the eyes.

## TEST PROCEDURE

*The Dose and Dose-Response Considerations*   Most household products should be tested in the form contained in their original package. When ocular contact with the packaged form is unlikely, the product should be tested in the form most likely to contact the eye.

With few exceptions[14] eye test methods have called for the instillation of 0.1 g or 0.1 ml of a material into the eye of the test animal. Although these quantities may be splashed around the eye, the amount of material that actually contacts ocular tissue in most accidents is probably considerably less. Indeed, the contrast between the severe effects in animal eye tests and the rarity of eye injuries in accidental human exposures to some classes of products may be as much a dose-response as a species-response phenomenon. Because the amount contacting the eye may be as important as the composition in determining the ocular response, there seems to be no basis for using a single, arbitrary dose in an eye test. Rather, two or more different doses would generate more information and permit the determination of dose-response characteristics of a material. The size of the doses and the difference between them should be determined partly by the physical characteristics of the test material. They should fall within the range of probable human exposure.

The measurement of the dose will depend on the physical form of the substance to be tested. Liquids and pastes can be delivered from a micropipette or syringe. Finely divided solids should be weighed to determine the amount equal to that contained in a specified volume when the material is lightly compacted. Other solids should be pulverized and then measured as above. Aerosol products should be delivered as a short, precisely timed burst at a distance approximating that of a self-inflicted eye exposure. For each dose form, the actual dose weight should be determined by weighing the same or an equal volume of the material. Suggested doses are 0.1 and 0.05 ml, though other volumes may be desirable when the range of human exposure is known or can be estimated.

The desired dose should be applied to the eye in a manner that reflects the probable route of accidental exposure. Whereas the instillation into the lower conjunctival cul-de-sac, as is customary with the Draize procedure, may be appropriate for drugs and cosmetics intended for use in and around the eye, the accidental exposure to other consumer products more often involves a speck, droplet, or spray on the lids or the bulbar surface. Furthermore, though the loose-fitting lower lid of the rabbit eye facilitates its use as a chamber to receive instilled materials, this technique is practically impossible to use with the monkey. In addition, it does not represent typical human exposure, as it tends to retain materials within the lids and in contact with the eye. For uniformity of technique, the lids should be drawn back and the material instilled directly onto the cornea. Great care should be taken to ensure that the entire dose is instilled onto the cornea. One of the greatest potential sources of experimental variation is incomplete dosage caused by movement by the animal or the technician. The lids should be kept open momentarily to ensure contact of the substance with the cornea, then gently released. Forced blinking or other manipulation that might cause trauma should be avoided. Self-trauma by the animals immediately after instillation should be prevented, as this will complicate evaluation of any toxic effect.

A single dose is administered to one eye of each animal in a test group. From three to six eyes have been specified in standard tests. Fewer eyes per dose should be needed when testing two or more dose levels than if a single level is used. A minimum of four animals may be used per dose level unless a smaller number will provide unequivocal evidence of severe irritation or corrosion. If there are large intragroup variations in response or inconsistent results between groups, an effort should be made to determine the cause (e.g., dosing error, reading error) and the test should be repeated.

*Irrigation*   Epidemiological evidence suggests that most eye accident victims rinse their eyes with water within 1 min of the exposure.[63] Certainly most physicians recommend prompt irrigation for accidental exposures to chemical substances with the rationale that the chemical on the surface is diluted and irrigated away. Nevertheless, experimental animal studies using the FHSA method[24,57] indicate that irrigation may decrease the amount of irritation caused by a chemical but is not likely to change an apparent irritant to a nonirritant. With some chemicals (1 percent sodium hydroxide), irrigation markedly diminishes the toxic effects. With 5 percent sulfuric acid, irrigation exacerbates the reaction.[60] The variability of irrigation techniques and the arbitrary nature of any one regimen further complicate a complex test without providing much useful information. For these reasons, irrigation is not a recommended requirement for any test for the inherent irritancy of a substance. Information on the effect of irrigation should be obtained with separate experimental groups. Such an investigation could be useful in determining appropriate first aid measures for use with materials that are corrosive or severely irritating.

*Controls and Comparison Standards*   Interlaboratory and temporal variability in rabbit eye testing[67] makes it difficult to determine the accuracy of any given result. Assuming that the factors that cause variability consistently affect all observations in a single test, it should be possible to compensate for them. This is done by testing control materials of established ocular irritancy and by rating unknown substances with respect to them. If the human response of the control material is known, animal response can be extrapolated to potential human response. In such cases, the more nearly alike the test material and control are in irritancy, the more confidence can be placed in extrapolation.

There are several criteria for the selection of an ideal control substance:

- Data on human experience should be available.
- Its composition should be known and its identity verifiable.
- Its physical and chemical properties should resemble those of the material to be evaluated.
- It should be readily obtainable in stable or reproducible condition.
- It should have similar dose-response characteristics to the test material.

*Observation Period*   If healing of the cornea and conjunctiva follow chemical injury, it is usually completed within 14 days. Nevertheless, a significant proportion of animals can show healing with clearing of the cornea after 14 days. Therefore, observation for 21 days is essential in any test for toxicity. Observations within the first 24 h may be of some value, but are not essential for most materials. If undertaken they should minimize manipulation of the eye and should not involve irrigation. Often the cornea may still be clear at 1 h but may later manifest severe changes. The recommended times for observations are 1, 3, 7, 14, and 21 days, though slight deviations from this schedule should not seriously affect results.

## STRUCTURE TO BE EVALUATED AND TOXIC EFFECTS

*Cornea*   The cornea is an important structure to evaluate. It is sensitive to chemicals; it is susceptible because of its prominence; and if damaged its structure often leads to impairment of vision. The extent of corneal damage is dependent on the nature of the material tested and the degree of exposure. Some chemicals may only damage the corneal epithelium or its superficial layers. Detection of only superficial epithelial damage may be very difficult without the use of the slit lamp or fluorescein staining. With only external observation and the use of some magnification, the cornea appears to "lack luster." With the slit lamp, a mild degree of edema of the epithelium can usually be seen. Superficial epithelial damage is best detected by staining with fluorescein. Where the superficial layers have been damaged, there is adsorption of fluorescein. This can be seen readily with or without a slit lamp.

More severe damage may cause the corneal epithelium to become detached and portions of it to roll up or become clumped on the corneal surface after 1 h. When the epithelium is detached, the cornea may be still clear after 1 h and there is usually no fluorescein staining. The absence of the corneal epithelium may be detected only with the slit lamp.

Superficial corneal epithelial damage in a small area usually clears after 1 to 3 days. When the entire corneal epithelium is denuded, healing is usually complete by 3 to 7 days. Before healing is complete, edema (thickening of the cornea) may occur. Subtle edema may only be apparent by the slit lamp. Epithelialization takes place peripherally in a centripetal fashion. The advanced edge of epithelium may have a slightly elevated appearance and is often edematous after irrigation. As the epithelium grows, it may have some melanin pigment, particularly in monkeys. This type of pigmentation is simply a sign of healing and does not necessarily indicate severity of damage.

With more severe reaction, the corneal stroma, in addition to the epithelium, is damaged. This usually results in edema of the cornea. The outcome depends on the intensity and extent of damage. Some lesions will clear; others may develop scarrings; and still others may lead to perforation of the cornea.

In general, acid compounds cause surface coagulation and are less likely to induce deeper tissue damage. Basic compounds have a greater predilection to diffuse and to penetrate into the tissues, thereby producing deep tissue damage.

*Iris*   Damage to the iris is difficult to detect. When there is direct chemical damage to the iris, the cornea becomes edematous. This obscures the details of the iris. When there is less severe damage to the cornea and conjunctiva, the iris may show some changes that, in part, may be due to neural reflexes.

In the albino rabbit these changes include vascular congestion, which gives the iris a reddish appearance as compared with its normal light-pink color. With more marked response the iris may become edematous with thickening and loss of the rugal pattern. Iris vessels may leak and give rise to inflammatory cells and increased amounts of protein in the aqueous humor.

These changes in the aqueous humor can be detected only with a slit lamp. The inflammatory cells can be observed directly and the protein noted by the Tyndall effect. In eyes with severe damage, the iris may give rise to intraocular bleeding.

*Conjunctiva and Nictitating Membranes*    The conjunctiva is a loosely arranged connective tissue that has an abundance of blood and lymph vessels. It is covered by nonkeratinized epithelium that is susceptible to only minimal damage compared to that described above for the cornea. When severely damaged, the vessels dilate, leak serum, and may even bleed. The vascular changes are responsible for the redness and swelling that follow chemical injury. Proteinaceous material from the serum and inflammatory cells form the ensuing exudate. Fluorescein is generally adsorbed by the conjunctiva following injury or total loss of the conjunctival epithelium and may be helpful in evaluating the effects after 1 to 3 days. Fluorescein is of less value in assessing severe damage. Extreme edema is observed with more severely toxic substances and with some that are not so toxic. In rabbits, for example, silver nitrate is particularly prone to inducing prominent conjunctival edema that is disproportionate to corneal damage.

More severe damage to the conjunctiva may be accompanied by scarring with distortion and folding of the conjunctiva. These folds may cover a portion of the corneal periphery. The nictitating membrane of rabbits is frequently damaged by chemical exposures, and, like the conjunctiva, it may become injected and edematous. Necrosis and scarring may be observed following more severe damage. Swelling of the conjunctiva may be so intense as to make evaluation of the cornea very difficult. Generally, when this occurs severe corneal damage can be observed once the edema has subsided.

At 7, 14, and 21 days after exposure to substances with lesser degrees of toxicity, there may be small superficial corneal opacities at the limbus after irrigation. By slit lamp these areas appear slightly edematous. These opacities are caused by mild neutrophilic infiltration within the corneal epithelium that is associated with similar infiltrates in the stroma and epithelium of the conjunctiva in the same meridian. This mild conjunctivitis may often be overlooked if histopathologic examination is not conducted.

When an eye with extreme, obviously purulent exudate at 7, 14, or 21 days is encountered, the animal should be handled carefully. One should avoid contact with the purulent exudate. If contact is made, one's hands should be washed before the next animal is touched. An obviously infected animal should be treated with an appropriate antibiotic by intramuscular injection. When care is not taken, the infection can be transmitted to other animals.

*Lids* The lid may become swollen following chemical injury. This causes the lids to become very tight, making evaluation of the eye difficult. With severe damage to the lids, the cilia (lashes) and hair of the lid may be lost. At 14 and 21 days the lid margin may be distorted with nicking as the result of scarring. With severe damage, as with 5 percent and 10 percent sodium hydroxide, the lids become severely scarred and fused together at 14 and 21 days. Perforation of the cornea is often associated with severe lid damage, although it may be masked by the fused lids.

SCORING OF LESIONS: DRAIZE PROCEDURE

By scoring of lesions one attempts to quantitate the area and degree of damage to the lids, conjunctiva, cornea, and interior of the eye. Lower numbers are given for smaller areas and intensity of damage; higher numbers are given to larger areas and greater intensities of damage. All methods require that the person examining the eyes and grading the lesions have considerable experience. Examinations should not be rushed, so that the lesions are not overlooked. The past standard method used for scoring ocular lesions was developed by Draize *et al.*[18] This method should be used in conjunction with bright illumination and some form of magnification.

The Draize method has the advantage of being relatively easy to conduct and requires little in the way of special equipment. The key to success with this method is the knowledge and experience of the examiner. There is now a considerable backlog of information using this method, though interlaboratory variation has been a problem. This is most likely due to different interpretation of lesions by different examiners.

*Cornea* Since damage to the cornea may lead to visual impairment, it is given special consideration. Corneal damage is determined by the presence of localized or diffuse opacification. Whether the iris details can be seen through the damaged area of the cornea is a factor considered in the quantitation of the corneal damage. Scattered or diffuse opacities that are only slight and allow for visualization of iris details are given a 1 rating. If the iris details are slightly obscured by easily discernible translucent areas of the cornea, a 2 rating is given. Opalescent areas of the cornea obscuring details of the iris and making the pupil barely discernible are given a 3 rating. If the iris is invisible through an opaque area of cornea, it is given a 4 rating.

The area of corneal damage is also quantitated. The scoring for percentages of corneal surface exhibiting any intensity opacity are: ≤ 25 percent = 1; > 25 percent but < 50 percent = 2; > 50 percent but < 75 percent = 3; and > 75 percent = 4.

While not considered in the original Draize scoring scheme, superficial and deep pannus (vascularization of the cornea) are noteworthy changes. Vascularization, which is part of the healing process, usually indicates that significant tissue necrosis has taken place. It can be rated by the intensity of associated opacification and by the area it affects, as above.

*Iris*    Evaluation of the iris is one of the most difficult aspects of the Draize method. If the cornea is relatively clear one can, with magnification, see the iris folds and note swelling, but these subtle changes are difficult to detect by this method.

The two more readily observed features of the iris are injection (color) and the pupillary light reflex. Congestion (redness) of the iris can be detected in the albino rabbit, but is not usually apparent in the monkey or pigmented rabbit.

With more marked corneal changes, the iris and even the pupillary light reflex may not be discernible. It is not clear how the iris is rated under these circumstances. If the iris cannot be adequately examined because of corneal changes, a maximal reading should probably be given, as histopathologic studies indicate iris damage in such cases.

The iris is rated 1 if any or all of the following are present even if pupillary light reflex is intact or only slightly impaired: more prominent iris folds, congestion, swelling, deep circumcorneal injection.

It is rated 2 if any or all of the following are observed: loss of pupillary reaction to light, hemorrhage in the interior of the eye, or obvious destruction of the iris.

*Conjunctiva*    Evaluation of the conjunctiva involves the quantitation of vascular congestion and hemorrhage (redness), edema (chemosis), and discharge (exudate).

Redness rating: 1—definite, but mild injection that causes a slight redness; 2—if injection is more diffuse, giving a more crimson-red appearance, and if individual vessels are not easily discernible; 3—if the conjunctiva has a diffuse, beefy-red appearance.

Chemosis rating: 1—slight swelling above normal; 2—obvious swelling with partial eversion of lids; 3—swelling with lids about half closed; 4—swelling with lids from about half closed to completely closed.

Exudate rating: 1—any amount of discharge different from normal; 2—discharge with moistening of the lids and adjacent hairs; 3—discharge with moistening of the lids and hairs for a considerable area around the eye.

*Totalling Scores*   The complete Draize grading scheme involves weighting of the corneal evaluation by multiplying opacity and area scores, then multiplying that product by 5. The iris score and the sum of the three conjunctival scores are weighted by factors of 5 and 2, respectively. The weighted scores can then be combined to give a maximum possible total of 110. There may be utility in this for some applications, but one should be aware that valuable information can be overlooked if too much emphasis is placed on a single number.

SCORING OF LESIONS: SLIT LAMP TECHNIQUE

The slit lamp used to observe ocular damage can accurately detect subtle lesions, but requires experience and careful judgment. It also requires that a second person hold the animal and coordinate with the biomicroscopist to expose various areas in succession.

The slit lamp projects a narrow beam of variable high-intensity light and has a binocular microscope that allows observation of the eye under magnification. Also the slit beam of light enables quantitation of the thickness of the cornea attributable to edema. Moreover, one can more clearly see the iris details and examine the aqueous humor in the anterior chamber for the presence of inflammatory cells and protein, both of which are signs of iritis.

The detection of changes in aqueous humor in the form of cellular reaction and presence of protein (aqueous flare or Tyndall effect) may be difficult, especially in eyes with more severely damaged corneas. Once the cornea becomes moderately thickened, it may not be possible to see these features. Vascular congestion of the iris and pupillary light reflex changes are more easily detected, even in eyes with moderate corneal thickening.

A scoring system for slit lamp observation also takes into account both the area and intensity of damage. This system emphasizes corneal edema and is determined by corneal thickness. The examiner must have a firm mental picture of the normal cornea and must repeatedly compare damaged, thickened areas with normal areas of the same eye or with the normal control eye.

*Cornea*   Evaluation of the corneal damage involves the determination of the presence of edema, fluorescein staining and subsequent scarring, vascularization, and perforation.

The intensity of corneal damage is rated 1 if there is only epithelial edema with or without slight stromal edema; 2, if the thickness has increased to 1.5 times the normal; 3, if the thickness has increased to 2 times the normal; and 4, when the cornea is entirely opaque and the thickness can not be determined.

Rating of the area of corneal involvement is the same as in the Draize method.

Fluorescein staining of the cornea may have a punctate or confluent pattern. The percentage of corneal surface with punctate or confluent staining and the rating scores are: $\leq$ 25 percent = 1; > 25 percent but < 50 percent = 2; > 50 percent but < 75 percent = 3; and > 75 percent = 4.

Areas of corneal vascularization, scarring, and pigment migration or persistent corneal edema are rated on the basis of area involvement in the same manner as described above for fluorescein staining and edema. Scars can occur at any point in the cornea. Vascularization and pigment migration occur first, and perhaps only, at the periphery of the cornea. Therefore, rating of vascularization and pigment migration is based on the area of circumference involved: $\leq$ 25 percent = 1; > 25 percent but < 50 percent = 2; > 50 percent but < 75 percent = 3; and > 75 percent = 4.

Corneal perforation is given a rating of 4. The total maximal score is 20, and the individual total score is the sum of ratings for area and intensity of corneal edema, fluorescein staining, vascularization, scarring or pigment migration, and perforation.

*Iris*  Iritis is quantitated by examination of the aqueous humor noting iris hyperemia and the status of the pupillary light reflex. Cells in the anterior chamber are rated 1, 2, or 3 on the basis of whether there are a few, a moderate number, or many, respectively. Aqueous flare (Tyndall effect) is similarly rated in the three intensities. Iris hyperemia is quantitated into slight (1), moderate (2), and marked (3) categories.

A sluggish pupillary light reflex is rated 1, and an absent reflex is rated 2. The total maximal score possible is 11, and an individual score is the sum of the ratings for anterior chamber cells, flare, iris hyperemia, and evaluation of the pupillary light reflex.

*Conjunctiva*  Lids and conjunctival damage are quantitated by giving a slight (1), moderate (2), and marked (3) rating for hypermia, chemosis, fluorescein staining, ulceration, and scarring. The total maximal score is 15. An individual score is the sum of all the ratings.

*Totalling Scores*  The total maximal slit lamp score is 46. The total individual score of any one reading is the sum of all the ratings for the cornea, iris, lid, and conjunctiva. Although slit lamp examination presents somewhat more difficulty for screening large numbers of materials, its use would seem to be indicated when evaluation of minimal dose effects is required. A slit lamp technique could also be employed in resolving questionable results by other techniques (e.g., Draize scoring).

*Use of Fluorescein*   Sodium fluorescein is a fluorescent dye that is helpful in detecting defects in the surface epithelium of the cornea and conjunctiva. With damage of the superficial layers of the epithelium, the dye is readily taken up by the remaining deeper layers and will fluoresce when light is cast on the area. With total loss of the corneal epithelium, fluorescein uptake on short contact with the dye is inconsistent at 1 day, but any significant lesions that might be missed or rated lower by the Draize method will be more clearly delineated. In most instances, lesions at 3, 7, 14, and 21 days are detected by gross observation without the use of fluorescein.

Fluorescein dye is available in two forms that are suitable for ocular testing. Sterile ophthalmologic solutions containing 0.25 percent to 1.0 percent sodium fluorescein are available commercially. Two drops of the solution are placed onto the cornea, then the animal is gently released. After 1 to 2 min, the fluorescein is irrigated out of the eye with 2 to 5 ml of saline or water. Sufficient irrigation is necessary to eliminate all excessive dye. The eye is then examined by the Draize method or by the slit lamp technique. Damaged areas adsorb the fluorescein dye and fluoresce in response to bright light. A cobalt-blue filter over the light source emphasizes the area of fluorescein staining, but is not essential in most instances. One must exert caution not to touch the eye with the dropper in order to prevent contamination of the dropper, the fluorescein solution, or the animals to be examined subsequently. New solutions should be used each day.

Fluorescein is also commercially available in individual, hermetically sealed paper strips. The fluorescein-containing end of a strip is moistened with two or three drops of water or saline, then gently applied to the conjunctiva so that some fluorescein drains onto the eye. A separate strip is used for each animal. The animal is released, the excess of fluorescein is irrigated away, and the eye is examined as above. The fluorescein paper strips have the advantage of reducing the chance of contamination.

EVALUATION

*Use of Optical Aids for Evaluation*   Any method to evaluate ocular damage should employ some means of magnification and good illumination. With the Draize technique, an operating lens loop is sufficient. The optimal instrument for both magnification and illumination is the slit lamp.

*Histopathological Examination*    This is an important aspect in any study where the quantitation of chemical damage is attempted. It is perhaps less vital in instances where obviously severe damage has occurred. Lesions that persist after exposure, at 21 days, however, may cause unwarranted higher ratings. The nature of such lesions becomes important. For example, the migration of pigment onto the cornea simply may represent the passive migration occurring as the result of the normal healing process of the corneal epithelium; however, other lesions may be scars and should be appropriately noted. Histopathological study may also disclose serious lesions of the conjunctiva and nictitating membrane that were not apparent or appreciated by examination with the Draize method or slit lamp technique.

It is desirable for an expert in screening substances to have knowledge of the histopathological alterations that account for such lesions. Green *et al.*[24] illustrate the clinical and histopathological features of various lesions at 1 h and at 1, 3, 7, 14, and 21 days in rabbits and monkeys. Their report also outlines techniques that maximize the chances of obtaining the clinically observed lesions in histological section.

*Photography*    Photographic documentation is an important aspect of ocular toxicity studies. While it is not essential in all series, any single laboratory involved with testing should build a reference library of photographs that is sufficient for teaching personnel to read ocular lesions. Such photographs can also be reviewed when there is interlaboratory variation in readings for specific substances. This double check on the examiner serves as a basis for correcting errors of judgment and technique. Photographs should be taken with equipment of sufficient quality to allow controlled exposures that will give close-up images in sharp focus, filling most of the camera field.

*Reversibility of Effects*    Whether or not toxic effects are reversible depends on the nature, extent, and intensity of damage. As noted above, most lesions, if reversible, will heal or clear within 21 days. Surface or epithelial damage is likely to heal with no residual abnormality. When large areas of epithelium are lost, healing takes longer. The epithelium that slides in from the periphery is very thin at first and may be associated with some edema. As the epithelium completely covers the denuded area, it regains its normal thickness and the edema disappears. Deep penetration by substances that induce stromal necrosis is more likely to be followed by scarring and vascularization. Once necrosis of the stroma of the cornea or conjunctiva occurs, then scarring takes place.

In some instances, especially after irrigation, persistent areas of peripheral corneal edema may be observed in an otherwise clear cornea. This may be due to residual inflammatory cells in the area of the edema or an associated area of residual conjunctivitis in the same meridian. Persumably this conjunctivitis and peripheral corneal edema clear with time.

*Classification of Responses*   The numerical scores for ocular responses as described above assist precise record-keeping and reporting. However, uncertainties about their quantitative significance and the differences among them make it desirable to have a more descriptive way of evaluating ocular responses. Furthermore, it is necessary to attach significance to persistence and reversibility of responses. The temporal aspect of injury as it might affect vision has the greatest implication for human safety.

Although the present FHSA eye test (16 CFR 1500.42; see Appendix A) does not include persistence of response as an evaluative criterion, the need for this is recognized. Methods have been suggested for factoring persistence of effects into the irritancy assessment;[3,30] however, their limited observation periods (from 3 to 7 days) are not long enough to establish the reversibility of some effects. By observing lesions for 3 wk, a more meaningful scale of severity can be developed. The following descriptive scale[24] is suggested for this purpose.

*Inconsequential or Complete Lack of Irritation*—Exposure of the eye to a material under the specified conditions causes no significant ocular changes. No staining with fluorescein can be observed. Any changes that occur clear within 24 h and are no greater than those caused by isotonic saline under the same conditions.

*Moderate Irritation*—Exposure of the eye to the material under the specified conditions causes minor, superficial, and transient changes of the cornea, iris, or conjunctiva as determined by external or slit lamp examination with fluorescein staining. The appearance at the 24-h or subsequent grading of any of the following changes is sufficient to characterize a response as moderate irritation: opacity of the cornea (other than a slight dulling of the normal luster), hyperemia of the iris, or swelling of the conjunctiva. Any changes that are seen clear within 7 days.

*Substantial Irritation*—Exposure of the eye to the material under the specified conditions causes significant injury to the eye, such as loss of the corneal epithelium, corneal opacity, iritis (other than a slight injection), conjunctivitis, pannus, or bullae. The effects clear within 21 days.

*Severe Irritation or Corrosion*—Exposure of the eye to the material under the specified conditions results in the same types of injury as in the previous category and in significant necrosis or other injuries that adversely affect the visual process. Injuries persist for 21 days or more.

Classification should be based on the most severe response seen in a group of test animals, rather than on the average response. If, however, one animal reacts with disproportionate severity so that the response seems spurious, the test should be repeated on at least four more eyes. If the response is not reproduced, a judgment can be made about whether it is appropriate to disregard it. Responses that are diminished in severity or persistence at the lowest test dose indicate that a material is less hazardous than one that produces slight or no change in response at a reduced dose. It follows that the smallest amount of a substance that will produce a substantial response may provide a useful index of its comparative irritancy. This scheme is still limited by the fact that it classifies responses in the test species only. These must then be extrapolated to probable human responses, as there is no appropriate experimental procedure for developing human ocular irritation data throughout the response scale. Extrapolations must be based on what is known about human experience, most of which is from accidental ocular exposures. This calls for the development of animal response information on control materials of known irritant or corrosive potential for humans. One or more control materials are tested simultaneously with the material being evaluated. The responses are then compared. To ensure optimum reliability of these comparisons, the controls and test substances should have similar properties, so that ocular responses will also be similar. Thus, one would not use sulfuric acid as a control in testing an alkaline material nor a water-soluble control in testing a hydrophobic material.

HUMAN TESTING

The predictability of animal eye test procedures is uncertain largely due to the dearth of reliable human dose-response data. Ethical considerations limit experiments with normal human eyes to those with transient and superficial toxic effects. This precludes a human testing to identify substances that might cause substantial or permanent changes in the eye, though it does not necessarily rule out the study of lesser ocular responses to determine thresholds and differences among species. Even then, such studies should be conducted only under the most scrupulous ethical standards and with fully informed consent of the subjects.

Advantage should be taken of any accidental human eye splashes of chemicals to establish some bases for comparison with animal data. These accidental eye splashes should be carefully recorded and reported in a manner as similar as possible to that used for the experimental procedure. Thorough characterization of the material involved should be included in the report.

## MUCOSAL IRRITATION AND CORROSION OF THE UPPER ALIMENTARY TRACT

Of particular importance is the ability to detect materials that, if ingested, can produce corrosive injury to the mucosal surfaces of the oral cavity, pharynx, esophagus, and stomach. Severe corrosive injury to these tissues can be fatal or can result in strictures or other permanent disabling injuries. Strong alkalis are likely to injure the esophagus and strong acids to injure the stomach and duodenum. Either may injure the tongue and pharynx.[64]

A provisional test method[50] is used by the Consumer Product Safety Commission,[7,54] but its reliability has not been established. In fact, there is no standardized procedure for predicting corrosive potential to the alimentary tract, though several techniques have been described. Materials have been administered by intraoral, intraesophageal, and intragastric gavage[9,16,39,49,70] and by timed application to specific tissues of solutions or impregnated tampons.[6,26,35,36] Rats, rabbits, cats, dogs, and swine have been tested, but a preferred animal model has not been identified.[41] The experts agree that more research is required before an animal model is selected and a reliable procedure is established.[60]

The need for a special test for esophageal corrosivity has been questioned[60] on the grounds that the customary battery of acute tests for oral toxicity, skin irritation, and eye irritation, when combined with information on chemical and physical properties, can provide reasonable presumptive evidence of a severe irritant or corrosive hazard on ingestion in the absence of empirical data. Indeed, the need for such an animal test might also be questioned on humane grounds.

## REFERENCES

1. Adams, E. M., D. D. Irish, H. C. Spencer, and V. K. Rowe. 1941. The response of rabbit skin to compounds reported to have caused acneform dermatitis. Ind. Med. 10(Ind. Hyg. Sect. vol. 2):1-4.
2. Bartek, M. J., J. A. LaBudde, and H. I. Maibach. 1972. Skin permeability *in vivo*: Comparison in rat, rabbit, pig and man. J. Invest. Dermatol. 58:114-123.
3. Bayard, S., and R. M. Hehir. 1976. Evaluation of proposed changes in the modified Draize rabbit eye irritation test. Presented at Society of Toxicology meeting, Atlanta, Ga., March 1976. Toxicol. Appl. Pharmacol. 37:186. Abstract no. 225.
4. Beckley, J. H. 1965. Comparative eye testing: Man *vs.* animal. Toxicol. Appl. Pharmacol. 2(Suppl.):93-101.
5. Beckley, J. H., T. J. Russell, and L. F. Rubin. 1969. Use of the rhesus monkey for predicting human response to eye irritants. Toxicol. Appl. Pharmacol. 15:1-9.
6. Berenson, M. M., and A. R. Temple. 1975. Detergent toxicity: Effects on esophageal and gastric mucosa. Clin. Toxicol. 8:399-404.
7. Bierbower, G. W., V. M. Seabaugh, J. R. Ferrell, and R. M. Hehir. 1973. Experimental

data taken from Consumer Product Safety Commission studies on the provisional esophageal rabbit test. Presented at the Soap and Detergent Association Invitational Symposium on Esophageal Corrosion Testing, Arlington, Va., Oct. 26, 1973.

8. Bleehen, S. S., M. A. Pathak, Y. Hori, and T. B. Fitzpatrick. 1968. Depigmentation of skin with 4-isopropylcatechol, mercaptoamines, and other compounds. J. Invest. Dermatol. 50:103-117.

9. Brown, N. M., and J. F. Griffith. 1974. Evaluation of non-phosphate detergent formulations for ingestion hazard. Toxicol. Appl. Pharmacol. 29:84. Abstract no. 23.

10. Buehler, E. V. 1965. Delayed contact hypersensitivity in the guinea pig. Arch. Dermatol. 91:171-177.

11. Buehler, E. V. 1974. Testing to predict potential ocular hazards of household chemicals. In: Winek, C. L., ed. Toxicology Annual 1974. New York, Marcel Dekker. pp. 53-69.

12. Buehler, E. V., and E. A. Newmann. 1964. A comparison of eye irritation in monkeys and rabbits. Toxicol. Appl. Pharmacol. 6:701-710.

13. Campbell, P., T. Watanabe, and S. K. Chandrasekaran. 1976. Comparison of in vitro skin permeability of scopolamine in rat, rabbit, and man. Fed. Proc. Fed. Am. Soc. Exp. Biol. 35:639. Abstract no. 2386.

14. Carpenter, C. P., and H. F. Smyth, Jr. 1946. Chemical burns of the rabbit-cornea. Am. J. Opthalmol. 29:1363-1372.

15. Carter, R. O., and J. F. Griffith. 1965. Experimental bases for the realistic assessment of safety of topical agents. Toxicol. Appl. Pharmacol. 2(Suppl.):60-73.

16. Cloyd, G. G., N. M. Brown, and J. F. Griffith. 1974. Methods for evaluating corrosive effects of ingesting detergents. Toxicol. Appl. Pharmacol. 29:83-84. Abstract no. 22.

17. Draize, J. H. 1959. Dermal toxicity. In: Association of Food and Drug Officials of the United States, Austin, Tex. Appraisal of the Safety of Chemicals in Foods, Drugs and Cosmetics. pp. 46-59.

18. Draize, J. H., G. Woodard, and H. O. Calvery. 1944. Methods for the study of irritation and toxicity of substances applied topically to the skin and mucous membranes. J. Pharmacol. Exp. Ther. 82:377-390.

19. Finkelstein, P., K. Laden, and W. Miechowski. 1965. Laboratory methods for evaluating skin irritancy. Toxicol. Appl. Pharmacol. 2(Suppl.):74-78.

20. Gaines, T. B. 1969. Acute toxicity of pesticides. Toxicol. Appl. Pharmacol. 14:515-534.

21. Gaines, T. B. 1960. The acute toxicity of pesticides to rats. Toxicol. Appl. Pharmacol. 2: 88-99.

22. Gellin, G. 1975. Prediction of human depigmenting chemicals with the guinea pig. In: Maibach, H. I., ed. Animal Models in Dermatology: Relevance to Human Dermatopharmacology and Dermatotoxicology. Edinburgh, Churchill Livingstone. pp. 267-272.

23. Grant, W. M. 1974. Toxicology of the Eye, 2d ed. Springfield, Ill., Charles C Thomas.

24. Green, W. R., J. B. Sullivan, R. M. Hehir, and L. G. Scharpf. 1976. A systematic comparison of chemically-induced eye injury in the albino rabbit and rhesus monkey. In: Soap and Detergent Association. Submission to the National Academy of Sciences by the Soap and Detergent Association on toxicity test procedures, with Appendices A-F. Appendix C.

25. Griffith, J. F., and E. V. Buehler. 1976. The prediction of skin irritancy and sensitizing potential by testing with animals and man. Presented at the Third Conference on Cutaneous Toxicity, Washington, D.C., May 16-18.

26. Haller, J. A., Jr., and K. Bachman. 1964. The comparative effect of current therapy on experimental caustic burns of the esophagus. Pediatrics 34:236-245.

27. Hunziker, N. 1969. Experimental Studies on Guinea Pig's Eczema. Their Significance in Human Eczema. New York, Springer-Verlag. pp. 31-36.

28. Jensen, N. E., I. B. Sneddon, and A. E. Walker. 1972. Tetrachlorobenzodioxin and chloracne. Trans. St. John's Hosp. Dermatol. Soc. 58:172-177.

29. Jones, E. L., and H. Krizek. 1962. A technic for testing acnegenic potency in rabbits, applied to the potent acnegen 2,3,7,8-tetrachlorodibenzo-*p*-dioxin. J. Invest. Dermatol. 39:511-517.
30. Kay, J. H., and J. C. Calandra. 1962. Interpretation of eye irritation tests. J. Soc. Cosmet. Chem. 13:281-289.
31. Klecak, G. 1977. Identification of contact allergens: Predictive tests in animals. *In*: Marzulli, F. N., and H. I. Maibach, eds. Dermatotoxicology and Pharmacology. Washington, D.C., Hemisphere Publishing Corp., distributed by Halsted Press, Division of John Wiley & Sons, New York. (Advances in Modern Toxicology, vol. 4.) pp. 305-340.
32. Kligman, A. M. 1966. The identification of contact allergens by human assay. III. The maximization test: A procedure for screening and rating contact sensitizers. J. Invest. Dermatol. 47:393-409.
33. Kligman, A. M., and W. Epstein. 1975. Updating the maximization test for identifying contact allergens. Contact Dermatitis 1:231-239.
34. Kligman, A. M., and W. M. Wooding. 1967. A method for the measurement and evaluation of irritants on human skin. J. Invest. Dermatol. 49:78-94.
35. Krey, H. 1952. On the treatment of corrosive lesions in the oesophagus; An experimental study. Acta Oto-Laryngol. 102(Suppl.):1-49.
36. Landau, G. D., and W. H. Saunders. 1964. The effect of chlorine bleach on the esophagus. Arch. Otolaryngol. 80:174-176.
37. Landsteiner, K., and J. Jacobs. 1935. Studies on the sensitization of animals with simple chemical compounds. J. Exp. Med. 61:643-656.
38. Lanman, B. M., W. B. Elvers, and C. S. Howard. 1968. The role of human patch testing in a product development program. Proc. Joint Conf. Cosmet. Sci., Washington, D.C., April 21-23. Washington, D.C., Toilet Goods Association. pp. 135-145.
39. Lee, J. F., D. Simonwitz, and G. E. Block. 1972. Corrosive injury of the stomach and esophagus by nonphosphate detergents. An experimental study. Am. J. Surg. 123:652-656.
40. McCreesh, A. H. 1965. Percutaneous toxicity. Toxicol. Appl. Pharmacol. 2(Suppl.):20-26.
41. MacDonald, W. E., A. G. Beasley, D. A. Cubit, and W. B. Deichmann. 1972. The acute oral toxicity and the hazard associated with the oral administration of two detergents. Ind. Med. Surg. 41(10):9-14.
42. MacMillan, F. S. K., R. R. Rafft, and W. B. Elvers. 1975. A comparison of the skin irritation produced by cosmetic ingredients and formulations in the rabbit, guinea pig, and beagle dog to that observed in the human. *In*: Maibach, H. I., ed. Animal Models in Dermatology: Relevance to Human Dermatopharmacology and Dermatotoxicology. Edinburgh, Churchill Livingstone. pp. 12-22.
43. Maguire, H. C., Jr. 1973. The bioassay of contact allergens in the guinea pig. J. Soc. Cosmet. Chem. 24:151-162.
44. Maibach, H. I. In press. Ten steps to percutaneous penetration. *In*: Chasseaud, L. F., ed. Progress in Drug Metabolism. London, John Wiley & Sons.
45. Maibach, H. I., G. Gellin, and M. Ring. 1975. Is the antioxidant butylated hydroxytoluene a depigmenting agent in man? Contact Dermatitis 1:295-296.
46. Maibach, H. I., and F. N. Marzulli. 1977. Phototoxicity (photoirritation) of topical and systemic agents. *In*: Marzulli, F. N., and H. I. Maibach, eds. Dermatotoxicology and Pharmacology. Washington, D.C., Hemisphere Publishing Corp., distributed by Halsted Press, Division of John Wiley & Sons, New York. (Advances in Modern Toxicology, vol. 4.) pp. 211-224.
47. Marzulli, F. N., and H. I. Maibach. 1975. The rabbit as a model for evaluating skin irritants: A comparison of results obtained on animals and man using repeated skin exposures. Food Cosmet. Toxicol. 13:533-540.

48. Marzulli, F. N., and H. I. Maibach. 1977. Contact allergy; predictive testing in humans. *In*: Marzulli, F. N., and H. I. Maibach, eds. Dermatotoxicology and Pharmacology. Washington, D.C., Hemisphere Publishing Corp., distributed by Halsted Press, Division of John Wiley & Sons, New York. (Advances in Modern Toxicology, vol. 4.) pp. 353-372.

49. Muggenburg, B. A., J. L. Mauderly, F. F. Hahn, S. A. Silbaugh, and S. A. Felicetti. 1974. Effects of the ingestion of various commercial detergent products by beagle dogs and pigs. Toxicol. Appl. Pharmacol. 30:134-148.

50. National Academy of Sciences-National Research Council. 1975. Principles for Evaluating Chemicals in the Environment. Report prepared for the Environmental Protection Agency by the Environmental Studies Board and the Committee on Toxicology. Washington, D.C. Oral irritation and corrosive effects, pp. 108-110.

51. Nixon, G. A., C. A. Tyson, and W. C. Wertz. 1975. Interspecies comparisons of skin irritancy. Toxicol. Appl. Pharmacol. 31:481-490.

52. Noakes, D. N., and D. M. Sanderson. 1969. A method for determining the dermal toxicity of pesticides. Br. J. Ind. Med. 26:59-64.

53. Odom, R. B., and H. I. Maibach. 1977. Contact urticaria: A different contact dermatitis. *In*: Marzulli, F. N., and H. I. Maibach, eds. Dermatotoxicology and Pharmacology. Washington, D.C., Hemisphere Publishing Corp., distributed by Halsted Press, Division of John Wiley & Sons, New York. (Advances in Modern Toxicology, vol. 4.) pp. 441-454.

54. Osterberg, R. E., G. W. Bierbower, V. M. Seabaugh, W. K. Porter, Jr., C. A. Hoheisel, and J. McLaughlin, Jr. 1976. Potential biological hazards of commercially available cleansers for artificial dentures. Toxicol. Appl. Pharmacol. 37:99-100. Abstract no. 18.

55. Phillips, L., II, M. Steinberg, H. I. Maibach, and W. A. Akers. 1972. A comparison of rabbit and human skin response to certain irritants. Toxicol. Appl. Pharmacol. 21:369-382.

56. Roudabush, R. L., C. J. Terhaar, D. W. Fassett, and S. P. Dziuba. 1965. Comparative acute effects of some chemicals on the skin of rabbits and guinea pigs. Toxicol. Appl. Pharmacol. 7:559-565.

57. Seabaugh, V. M., R. E. Osterberg, C. A. Hoheisel, J. C. Murphy, and G. W. Bierbower. 1976. A comparative study of rabbit ocular reactions to various exposure times to chemicals. Presented at Society of Toxicology meeting, Atlanta, Ga., March 1976. Toxicol. Appl. Pharmacol. 37:187. Abstract no. 227.

58. Shelanski, H. A., and M. V. Shelanski. 1953. A new technique of human patch tests. Proc. Sci. Sect. Toilet Goods Association. 19:46-49.

59. Shelley, W. B., and A. M. Kligman. 1957. The experimental production of acne by penta- and hexachloronaphthalenes. Arch. Dermatol. 75:689-695.

60. Soap and Detergent Association. 1976. Submission to the National Academy of Sciences by the Soap and Detergent Association on toxicity test procedures, with Appendices A-F. New York, SDA. Appendix F: Summary of SDA Invitational Symposium on Esophageal Corrosion held on October 26, 1973.

61. Steinberg, M., W. A. Akers, M. Weeks, A. H. McCreesh, and H. I. Maibach. 1975. A comparison of test techniques based on rabbit and human skin responses to irritants with recommendations regarding the evaluation of mildly or moderately irritating compounds. *In*: Maibach, H. I., ed. Animal Models in Dermatology: Relevance to Human Dermatopharmacology and Dermatotoxicology. Edinburgh, Churchill Livingstone. pp. 1-11.

62. Stoughton, R. B. 1975. Animal models for *in vitro* percutaneous absorption. *In*: Maibach, H. I., ed. Animal Models in Dermatology: Relevance to Human Dermatopharmacology and Dermatotoxicology. Edinburgh, Churchill Livingstone. pp. 121-132.

63. Temple, A. R., J. C. Veltri, and C. Gillies. 1976. Summary of potentially toxic eye exposures and the outcome of these exposures on the victim involving soaps, detergents and other

household care products for the period October 14, 1974, through October 14, 1975. *In*: Soap and Detergent Association. Submission to the National Academy of Sciences by the Soap and Detergent Association on toxicity test procedures, with Appendices A-F. Appendix D.1.

64. Tucker, A. S., and E. W. Gerrish. 1960. Hydrochloric acid burns of the stomach. J. Am. Med. Assoc. 174:890-893.
65. U.S. Food and Drug Administration. 1972. Hazardous substances: Proposed revision of test for primary skin irritants. Fed. Reg. 37(244):27635-27636, Dec. 19.
66. Weil, C. S., N. I. Condra, and C. P. Carpenter. 1971. Correlation of 4-hour vs. 24-hour contact skin penetration toxicity in the rat and rabbit and use of the former for predictions of relative hazard of pesticide formulations. Toxicol. Appl. Pharmacol. 18:734-742.
67. Weil, C. S., and R. A. Scala. 1971. Study of intra- and interlaboratory variability in the results of rabbit eye and skin irritation tests. Toxicol. Appl. Pharmacol. 19:276-360.
68. Wester, R. C., and H. I. Maibach. 1975. Percutaneous absorption in the rhesus monkey compared to man. Toxicol. Appl. Pharmacol. 32:394-398.
69. Wester, R. C., and H. I. Maibach. 1975. Rhesus monkey as an animal model for percutaneous absorption. *In*: Maibach, H. I., ed. Animal Models in Dermatology: Relevance to Human Dermatopharmacology and Dermatotoxicology. Edinburgh, Churchill Livingstone. pp. 133-137.
70. Williams, J. B., and D. Taber. 1972. Assessing detergent safety: A comparison of a nonphosphate laundry detergent with phosphate detergents. J. Am. Oil Chem. Soc. 49:539-551.

# 4 Inhalation Exposure

This chapter addresses that part of the *Federal Hazardous Substances Act Regulations* that define toxic substances as inhalation hazards [16 CFR 1500.3(b)(5) and (b)(6)(i)(B); see Appendix A]. Hazardous airborne substances are those that occur in concentrations that could foreseeably be encountered by humans during use. However, the methodologies discussed here should be able to assess potential toxicity caused by accidental inhalation of high concentrations, as well as low concentrations likely to be encountered over a long period. Thus, careful consideration has been given to inhalation tests and techniques that could serve as guidelines not only for assessment of acute inhalation toxicity, but also for subchronic and chronic toxicity. Assessment of chronic toxicity has assumed greater importance with the increased recognition of chronic toxic response.

This chapter will serve as a guideline for the conduct of inhalation toxicity assessment and be of assistance in determining procedures to be used in complying with the *Regulations*. It is not, however, meant to be an all-inclusive listing of methodologies used for total assessment of the inhalation hazard of potentially toxic substances, nor does it address inhalation toxicology in its entirety. Greater detail of testing methods can be found in the literature.[5]

Technological advances have resulted in a variety of potentially toxic household products. A host of these, known and unknown, can produce injury to tissue and body systems. The respiratory tract is particularly vulnerable to many substances, as it is generally less protected than most body systems.

60

Moreover, it can be subjected to insult, not only when a toxicant enters the body through the respiratory tissue, but also, in some instances, when a toxicant leaves the body via the respiratory tract after having gained entry by a different route. Consequently, injuries to lung and other body tissue resulting from inhaled toxic substances can have numerous ramifications, depending on the degree of toxicity of the substance, concentration and duration of exposure, and existence of an immediate or latent effect. The anatomy and physiology of the respiratory tract have great influence on the toxicity of inhaled vapors, gases, and particularly inhaled particles.

## EXPOSURE CHAMBERS

It is important to distinguish between aerosols and vapors or gases. The term "aerosol" usually refers to solid or liquid particulates but not gases or vapors that arise from liquid surfaces. But because gases and vapors may become adsorbed on particulate material, they may also be included with aerosols. In many household products, mixtures of solids, liquids, and vapors or gases may be present.

Gases can be metered from pressurized cylinders through calibrated flow meters fitted with differential pressure gauges to avoid the influence of pressure on flow. The gas flow is then mixed with the diluting stream of air or other gas at the same pressure. It is then led into the exposure chamber. Metering pumps are also used in the flow metering of gases or vapors from liquid surfaces. Vapors can be generated from certain liquids (b.p. 30°C-70°C) by metering the liquid onto a mildly heated surface, diluting the vapor with air, and then leading the mixture to the animal exposure chamber. Chamber concentrations should be determined. Thermal degradation at the site of vaporization should be avoided.

To prepare liquid and solid aerosols, the parent material should be broken up into particles of respirable diameter ($< 5 \mu$m). This permits the particle to navigate the tortuous passages of the respiratory tree and impact on the alveolar surfaces. The Wright dust feed mechanism, the Lovelace aerosol particle separator (for monodisperse aerosols), the Vaponephrin nebulizer (liquids), and the Laskin atomizer can be used for this purpose.[8,19,21]

Casarett and Doull[5] have classified particulate materials, discussed their behavior, and described the environmental factors that govern their characteristics. Aerodynamic particle size is the most important property of an aerosol with regard to its potential pulmonary deposition and toxic action. In general, the smaller the particle diameter, the deeper its penetration into the respiratory tract. The mass of the particle is also important toxicologically, because toxic effects are consistently related to the mass of the inhaled particles and the number of particles per unit volume of inspired air. Thus, the particle diameter and density govern aerodynamic behavior in the airstreams; mass determines the dosage and, consequently, the magnitude of the toxic effect.

Other factors to be considered are hygroscopicity, particle shape (e.g., fibrous), the total charge on the particle, and the density of the charge. In the humid environment of the respiratory tree, a hygroscopic particle will grow in size, thereby changing the deposition site and possibly the toxic effect.

When used as intended, household products in aerosol form are polydisperse, i.e., they have a wide range of particle sizes. Consequently, these size fractions are deposited at different sites in the respiratory tree. Though the numbers vary, particles between 5 and 30 $\mu$m in diameter impact because of inertial forces in the nasopharyngeal zone; particles from 1 to 5 $\mu$m in diameter deposit by sedimentation onto the tracheobronchial region; and particles $\leq$ 1 $\mu$m in diameter flow into the alveolar region. Because of this, the polydisperse aerosol from a household product, e.g., a material sprayed from a pressurized container, could have different toxic effects, depending on the impact zone as affected by the particle size mass distribution.

Within the exposure chamber the test agent is influenced by humidity, surface characteristics (lining material), temperature, and flow rate through the system. In inhalation exposure chambers, these factors should be stabilized. For example, when several groups of animals are exposed to the same product, the operating variables should be consistent among the chambers used. The chamber temperature and humidity should be controlled and monitored.

The nominal concentration of gas, vapor, or aerosol within the chamber can be computed from the amount delivered from the generator and the air flowing into the chamber. Flow rate and chamber size should be such that the uptake curve is sufficiently steep to reach the desired concentration promptly. Concentrations tested should not be so great as to reduce appreciably the available oxygen or to approach the lower explosive limit of flammable systems. Silver[20] has shown the pattern of chamber uptake of a gas in a dynamic exposure chamber. Analyses can be used to show this uptake pattern and demonstrate the maintenance concentration. Several analytical techniques are in use for chamber analyses. These include impactors for particulate aerosols, wet chemical methods, colorimetry, gas-liquid chromatography, atomic-absorption spectroscopy, infrared spectrophotometry, light-scattering particle counters, and other instrumental methods. It is technologically important that the nominal and analytical concentrations be close, because this indicates good control over loss of the test agent. If this principle is observed, analyses during the exposure period need not be frequent, thus resulting in a cost-effective operation.

Household products, especially polymeric ones, may be subjected to heat and undergo thermal degradation. The fumes generated by this heating could be irritating and possibly toxic. Standard methodology for evaluation of pyrolysis/combustion products is not yet available; however, the National Academy of Sciences has published guidelines.[17]

The complexity of toxicologic evaluation is compounded in the case of inhalation exposures, not only because of equipment requirements, but also because of questions of actual concentration inhaled and amount retained. The dosage depends on several factors, including physical and chemical properties of the agent, target tissue and kinetics of penetration, disposition, normal and/or impaired clearance mechanism, metabolic conversion, and the number of entry routes, e.g., skin and/or ingestion. Dosage and the amount entering the internal milieu of the body is difficult to determine for inhalation exposures. That is why inhalation toxicologists refer to exposure in lieu of dose. Exposure is defined in terms of concentration ($c$), time ($t$), and, sometimes, both ($ct$).[15]

There are many types of inhalation exposure chambers,[7,8] but general purpose units are sufficient for the exposures discussed in this chapter.

Inhalation systems are basically categorized into two types: static or dynamic. The static system introduces the test agent into the chamber as a batch, followed by mixing; the dynamic system has a continuous airflow and introduction of the test agent. Static systems have limitations, primarily the loss of exposure agent with consequent decrease in concentration. Also, the volume of the chamber poses a limitation because of oxygen depletion and carbon dioxide and heat buildup.

The exposure technique generally used today, and most appropriate to this chapter, uses dynamic systems in which both the airflow and introduction of the test agent(s) are continuous. The agent is introduced into the chamber until the concentration becomes constant and perfect mixing occurs. Then, the theoretical concentration can be calculated. The dynamics of such systems have been described and verified,[20] but many factors, such as flow variability, animal uptake, and adsorption to chamber walls and/or animals, contribute to a difference between theoretical and actual concentration in the exposure unit. Thus, there is need to measure the actual concentration by sampling and analysis. Otherwise, characterization of exposure concentration and dose-response relationship is questionable.

When exposing small numbers of animals, particularly in pilot tests and/or LC50 studies with rodents, exposure systems typically consist of a closed container with facilities for air and contaminant supply and exhaust. A simple version is the cylindrical battery jar (or all-glass chamber), which is small enough to be operated in a fume hood. A minimum size of 30 to 40 liters can accommodate 6 to 10 rats, depending upon age. Such units are described in

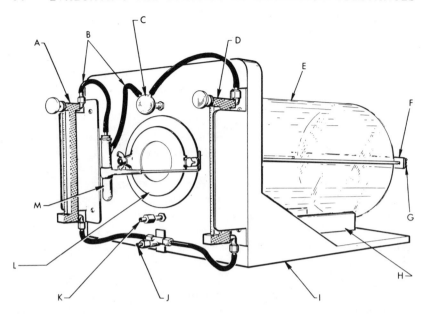

FIGURE 1    Schematic diagram of inhalation exposure unit. (A) Vapor generator rotameter; (B) nonreactive tubing; (C) mixing flask; (D) diluting air rotameter; (E) glass cylinder; (F) wooden clamping bar; (G) wing nut; (H) glass cylinder support; (I) wooden frame; (J) compressed air inlet; (K) chamber exhaust outlet; (L) door; (M) vapor generator. Adapted from Leach.[11]

detail elsewhere.[7,18] These are depicted in Figures 1 and 2. Because of the limitation imposed by chamber size, it may be difficult to adhere to the recommended practice of containing the animals in individual compartments within the exposure chambers.

A second small system, which lends itself to greater adaptability and utility in single and some repeated testing, was designed by Laskin and Drew[10] (see Figure 3). The chamber is a cylinder, 14 in. in diameter and 2 ft long, with domes at either end. It is supported by a plywood-metal frame. Standard rubber O-rings serve as gaskets between the cylinder and the domes. Plastic fittings are cemented to the domes and act as intake and exhaust ports. The lower dome is permanently mounted, while the upper dome is removable to provide access for animal cages. This system is comparatively inexpensive and can be replaced if contaminated or affected by test agents.

"Rochester" or "New York University" inhalation chambers (Figures 4 and 5), or modifications thereof, are generally regarded as the systems of choice for repeated exposures.[7,12] These are used in a great number of inhalation facilities. The bodies of the chambers are made of stainless steel with

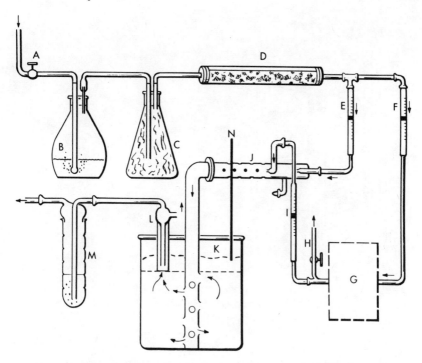

FIGURE 2   Schematic diagram of composite inhalation glass exposure unit. (A) Reducing valve on compressed air inlet; (B) potassium dichromate-sulfuric acid cleaning solution; (C) glass wool filter system; (D) dessicant; (E) rotameter for dilution air; (F) rotameter for contaminant pickup; (G)contaminant source; (H) contaminant (agent-air) bleed-off; (I) rotameter to monitor contaminant supply; (J) mixing tube; (K) exposure line; (L) exhaust line; (M) sampling tube connected to vacuum source; (N) thermometer.

windows and are available in various sizes. The toxicant is supplied into the clean airstream at the top of the chamber. Both animal wastes and air are removed at the bottom of the pyramid, the air going up the side arm of a **Y** fitting at the bottom of the chamber. A valve and/or trap in the bottom maintains the static pressure of the system, as well as preventing sewer gas, vermin, etc., from entering the chamber.

Design and/or operation of inhalation systems demand good engineering principles. The airflow through the chambers varies from 10 to 60 air changes per hour, the lower limit being a function of heat removal and maintenance of oxygen/carbon dioxide balance for a total animal volume usually not greater than 5 percent of the total chamber volume. Dynamic chambers have air-exchange rates that are exponential. A flow-through of air equal to the volume of a chamber does not even approach a complete air exchange.[15]

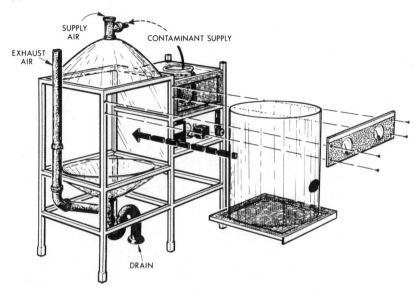

FIGURE 3    Schematic diagram of plastic exposure chamber.

Airflow is monitored with venturi and/or orifice meters.[9] Accurate construction, calibration, and placement of such devices are important factors. Intake air should be filtered with absolute filters and/or charcoal filters before introduction into the chamber with the test agent. It is particularly important to assure that the airborne agent is removed from the air prior to exhausting it into the atmosphere. Filter systems must be selected judiciously. Scrubbers or charcoal absorbers should be used in the exhaust process. Filters, electrostatic precipitators, cyclones, or a combination of these will remove particulates from air leaving the chamber. The importance of these factors can be readily appreciated if the substance being tested happens to be a suspected carcinogen. The selection of exhaust air-cleaning systems should be based on the pollutant in question. The effluent air should be monitored to check on the efficiency of the air-cleaning process. Detailed studies of such considerations should be consulted.[7,8]

Temperature and humidity should be monitored by remote probes with either continuous recording devices or visual display.[8,13] Static pressure within the chamber should be measured with a Magnehelic gauge in order to maintain a slightly negative pressure. Whenever possible, fail-safe devices should be built into the generation system to prevent accidental overexposure.[22] This precautionary measure could save the experiment in the event of a power failure, as the test agent would not otherwise be stopped during loss of airflow through the chamber.

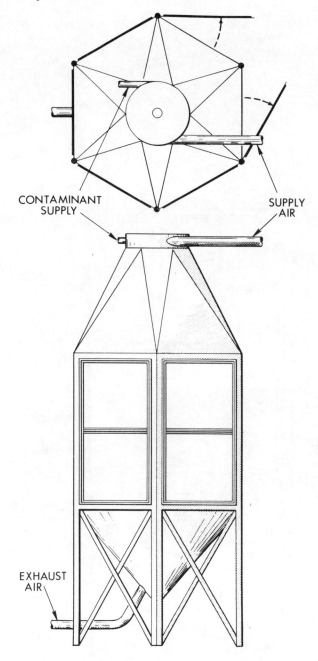

CONTAMINANT
SUPPLY

SUPPLY
AIR

EXHAUST
AIR

FIGURE 4   Schematic diagram of the "Rochester" exposure chamber.

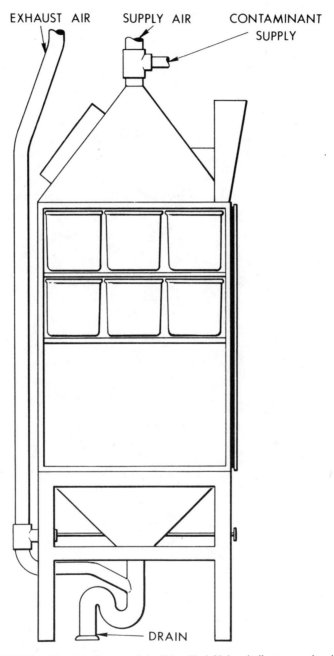

FIGURE 5   Schematic diagram of the "New York University" exposure chamber.

In several situations it is desirable to expose only the head or the nose of the test animals; for example, when skin and/or ingestion could complicate interpretation of the effects of the test agents. Good toxicological evaluation demands innovative techniques.[7]

## ACUTE INHALATION EXPOSURES

Single, high-concentration, inhalation exposures are used to determine the approximate toxicity level of a chemical compound or mixture for comparative purposes. Broad classification levels are defined in 16 CFR 1500.3 (see Appendix A). The nature of the toxic effect, if any, should also be determined through this process. The concentrations to be used in chronic repeated inhalation exposure tests can be established. These procedures are also applicable to brief and intermittent human exposures.

The most informative and useful technique for determining the acute toxic effects of inhalation exposure is the one used to determine the LC50 value for rats. An LC50 value is that atmospheric concentration statistically estimated to kill 50 percent of the animals exposed for a fixed time within a specified postexposure period. Title 21 of the *Code of Federal Regulations* defines the exposure period as 1 h and the observation period as 14 days.

Using the contaminant-generation techniques and chambers described earlier, rats weighing between 200 and 300 g are exposed in groups of 6 to 10 animals each to several measured air concentrations and observed for 14 days. The statistical confidence limits will vary with the number of animals. When it is determined that at least three groups have 14-day mortality rates between 16 percent and 85 percent, the LC50 value and its 95 percent confidence limits can be calculated using the method of Litchfield and Wilcoxon[14] or Miller and Tainter.[16]

Preliminary range-finding tests can be conducted using two or three animals in each group. Exposures should begin with a relatively high concentration (e.g., 10,000 ppm). If 100 percent mortality is achieved within 1 h, succeeding test concentrations should be reduced by a factor of 10 until no deaths occur during the specified period. At this point a judgment can be made concerning the concentrations to be used in the LC50 study based on severity or lack of toxic signs observed in the range-finding tests.

Although death is the measured end point for the LC50 determination, observation of toxic signs should be made and recorded. The types of observations and records to be made are described in previous chapters. Animals exposed via the inhalation route should be observed for at least 2 h postexposure for signs of irritation of eyes, nose, and lung tissue. Gross changes in respiratory rate, diaphragmatic breathing or gasping, and frothing or bleeding from the nares are some signs of irritation of lung tissue. Other evidence of discomfort may be pawing at the eyes or nose. In addition to these observations, records should include time of death and gross pathological changes noted at necropsy.

## CHRONIC EXPOSURE STUDIES

Repeated inhalation exposures are conducted with products whose intended use will be frequent and for extended periods. For purposes of these guidelines, the number of repeated exposures to be conducted depends on the purposes of the experiment and the use of the product (e.g., 2 days up to a lifetime). The terms subchronic or chronic have been used to describe these studies.

### TEST DESIGN

The number of animals to be used in each group should be determined by length of the experiment and the observations, measurements, and interim sacrifices to be made during the exposure periods. At least one rodent and one nonrodent species should be used for all repeated exposure studies. The laboratory rat is the rodent of choice, and, depending on the available chamber size and configuration, either the nonhuman primate or the dog is the nonrodent species of choice.

The minimum number of animals for the various periods of study are shown in Table 1. In studies longer than 1 yr, the initial weight of the rats should range from 50 to 75 g (weanlings). Shorter studies should begin with rats weighing from 100 to 150 g. The number of nonrodents in each experimental and control group should provide at least four males and four females for pathological evaluation at the end of the study. Dogs should be between 4 and 6 mo of age; nonhuman primates should be young adults.

TABLE 1    Minimum No. of Animals to Be Used in Different Exposure Periods

| Group No. | Exposure | Rats | | | | | | Nonrodents | |
|---|---|---|---|---|---|---|---|---|---|
| | | < 10 days | | 10-180 days | | > 180 days | | All Exposure Periods | |
| | | Male | Female | Male | Female | Male | Female | Male | Female |
| I. | Control filtered air | 10 | 10 | 20 | 20 | 50 | 50 | 4 | 4 |
| II. | Low level | 10 | 10 | 20 | 20 | 50 | 50 | 4 | 4 |
| III. | Intermediate level | 10 | 10 | 20 | 20 | 50 | 50 | 4 | 4 |
| IV. | High level | 10 | 10 | 20 | 20 | 50 | 50 | 4 | 4 |

The length of each daily exposure and the duration of the study should be determined by the intended use of the product. For example, the intended use of some products is once a day for a very short duration (minutes); with others, such as paint vapors, the exposure may be for hours. Therefore, the daily duration of exposure of animals in a repeated-exposure study should approximate the exposure conditions of the product user. Simulation of actual use conditions is not always advised as an initial step, as controlled studies at an effect level can sometimes give information that will more clearly delineate the desired levels for repeated exposures over long periods.

The following observations should be made and recorded during the exposure:

• *Clinical signs.* Each animal should be observed twice daily for signs of toxicity.

• *Body weights.* The body weights of the rats should be recorded initially, weekly during the first 13 wk, and monthly thereafter. Body weights of the nonrodents should be recorded initially and monthly throughout the study.

• *Hematology and clinical biochemistry studies.* Hematology and clinical studies should be conducted prior to and periodically throughout the exposure in the nonrodent species. For practical reasons, clinical biochemistry studies may be limited to times of sacrifice and the end of the exposure period for the rats. The types of measurements should be determined, if possible, from prior knowledge of the toxicity of the product, such as signs that were manifested during preliminary short-term toxicity tests. Certain measurements serve as an index of the health status of the laboratory animals (see Appendix C for suggested list). The importance of quality control cannot be overemphasized. It is imperative that clinical laboratories participate in a quality-control program.


PATHOLOGY STUDIES

*Gross Pathology and Tissue Fixation*   Each animal that dies, as well as all survivors, should be necropsied and all gross lesions noted. A careful examination of all organs should be made by trained technicians who are supervised by competent animal pathologists. After select organs are removed at necropsy and weighed, the ratios of organ to terminal body weight may be calculated (see Appendix D for suggested list). The major organs and tissues should be removed at necropsy and fixed in 10 percent neutral buffered formalin (see Appendix D for suggested list). The lung should be removed *in*

72    EVALUATING THE TOXICITY OF HOUSEHOLD SUBSTANCES

*toto* and perfused intratracheally with an amount of 10 percent neutral buffered formalin that is equal to approximately 75 percent of the total lung capacity (TLC) for that species. A maximum pressure of 25 cm of water should be used for perfusion.

*Histopathology*    Microscopic slides of the tissues should be prepared and evaluated from all animals in the control and high-level groups. Sections from all lobes of the lung should be examined. In the low- and intermediate-exposure groups, histopathological examination should be made of at least the nasal cavity, lungs, trachea, peribronchial lymph nodes, liver, kidneys, gonads, and all grossly observed lesions. Any others that showed injury in the high-exposure group should also be examined for the low and intermediate groups.

*Statistical Analysis*    Appropriate statistical tests should be applied to the body weight, organ weight, and organ/body weight ratios.

SPECIAL LABORATORY TECHNIQUES

There are many special laboratory techniques available for evaluating the toxicity of inhaled household products. These include intratracheal administration, pulmonary clearance studies of the rate of removal of particles from the respiratory tract, alveolar macrophage studies to assess the response to irritant materials,[4,6] body plethysmographic studies to determine sensory response,[1,2] and pulmonary flow-resistance studies.[3] While it may be desirable to use these techniques in some situations, they generally require special equipment and experience and are not recommended for routine application.

CARCINOGENICITY STUDIES

When planning a carcinogenicity experiment by the inhalation route, refer to Chapter 5 for experiment design.

## REFERENCES

1. Alarie, Y. 1966. Irritating properties of airborne materials to the upper respiratory tract. Arch. Environ. Health 13:433-449.
2. Alarie, Y. 1973. Sensory irritation by airborne chemicals. CRC Crit. Rev. Toxicol. 2:299-363.
3. Amdur, M. O., and J. Mead. 1958. Mechanism of respiration in unanesthetized guinea pigs. Am. J. Physiol. 192:364-368.

4. Brain, J. D. 1970. Free cells in the lungs: Some aspects of their role, quantitation, and regulation. Arch. Intern. Med. 126:477-487.

5. Casarett, L. J., and J. Doull, eds. 1975. Toxicology: The Basic Science of Poisons. New York, Macmillan.

6. Coffin, D. L., D. E. Gardner, R. S. Holzman, and F. J. Wolock. 1968. Influence of ozone on pulmonary cells. Arch. Environ. Health 16:633-636.

7. Drew, R. T., and S. Laskin. 1973. Environmental inhalation chambers. *In*: Gay, W. I., ed. Methods of Animal Experimentation, vol. 4. New York, Academic Press. pp. 1-41.

8. Fraser, D. A., R. E. Bales, M. Lippmann, and H. E. Stokinger. 1959. Exposure Chambers for Research in Animal Inhalation. Public Health Monograph no. 57. Public Health Service publ. no. 662. Washington, D.C., Government Printing Office.

9. Hinners, R. G., J. K. Burkart, and C. L. Punte. 1968. Animal inhalation exposure chambers. Arch. Environ. Health 16:194-206.

10. Laskin, S., and R. T. Drew. 1970. An inexpensive portable inhalation chamber. Am. Ind. Hyg. Assoc. J. 31:645-646.

11. Leach, L. J. 1963. A laboratory test chamber for studying airborne materials. Atomic Energy Commission Research and Development Report UR-629. Rochester, N.Y., University of Rochester. pp. 1-12.

12. Leach, L. J., C. J. Spiegl, R. H. Wilson, G. E. Sylvester, and K. E. Lauterbach. 1959. A multiple chamber exposure unit designed for chronic inhalation studies. Am. Ind. Hyg. Assoc. J. 20:13-22.

13. Lee, D. H. K. 1964. Heat and Cold Effects and Their Control. Public Health Monograph No. 72. Public Health Service Publication No. 1084. Washington, D.C., Government Printing Office.

14. Litchfield, J. T., Jr., and F. Wilcoxon. 1949. A simplified method of evaluating dose-effect experiments. J. Pharmacol. Exp. Ther. 96:99-113.

15. MacFarland, H. N. 1968. Design and operation of exposure chambers. Proceedings of the 7th Annual Technical Meeting of the American Association for Contamination Control, Chicago. pp. 19-25.

16. Miller, L. C., and M. L. Tainter. 1944. Estimation of the ED50 and its error by means of logarithmic-probit graph paper. Proc. Soc. Exp. Biol. Med. 57:261-264.

17. National Academy of Sciences-National Research Council, Committee on Fire Toxicology. 1977. Fire Toxicology: Methods for Evaluation of Toxicity of Pyrolysis and Combustion Products; Report no. 2. Washington, D.C.

18. National Academy of Sciences-National Research Council, Committee on Toxicology. 1964. Principles and Procedures for Evaluating the Toxicity of Household Substances. Washington, D.C. NAS Publication No. 1138.

19. Raabe, O. G., G. M. Kanapilly, and G. J. Newton. 1971. New methods for the generation of aerosols of insoluble particles for use in inhalation studies. *In*: Walton, W. H., ed. Inhaled Particles III, vol. 1. Surrey, England, Unwin Brothers Ltd. pp. 3-18.

20. Silver, S. D. 1946. Constant flow gassing chambers: Principles influencing design and operation. J. Lab. Clin. Med. 31:1153-1161.

21. Talley, D., O. G. Raabe, and J. A. Mewhinney. 1975. Lovelace aerosol particle separator design modifications. *In*: Inhalation Toxicology Research Institute, Annual Report 1974-1975. Albuquerque, N.M., Lovelace Foundation for Medical Education and Research. U.S. Energy Research and Development Administration report no. LF-52. pp. 24-27.

22. Thomas, A. A. 1965. Chamber equipment design considerations for altitude exposures. Proc., Conference on Atmospheric Contamination in Confined Spaces. Wright-Patterson Air Force Base, Ohio. AMRL-TR-65-230. pp. 9-17.

# 5 Chronic Toxicity/Carcinogenicity Tests

The ideal chronic toxicity test in animals should reliably predict all of the potential health hazards that might be associated with a long-term, low-level exposure of man to a toxic agent. Although negative findings in such tests are frequently used to establish safety (or safe exposure levels), the primary goal of the chronic toxicity test, like that of all toxicity tests in animals, is to identify and characterize toxicity. Since its purpose is to detect injury in all target organs and systems, its protocols may differ appreciably from those for tests designed to detect specific toxic effects, such as carcinogenesis or teratogenesis. Although information about the carcinogenic potential of a toxic agent may be obtained from a well-designed chronic study, these tests provide more information than a simple carcinogenesis bioassay. Similarly, the use of combined protocols to obtain information about the teratogenic, reproductive, behavioral, and other effects of an agent as a dividend of these tests may impose levels and duration constraints that destroy the original purpose of the chronic test.

In addition to detecting the chronic toxic effects of a chemical, such studies should also identify the exposure levels that produce the injury, as well as those that produce no observed effects. Chronic toxicity tests should provide, therefore, data on both the dose-effect and dose-response characteristics of the chemical under study. The classical approach to the study of chronic toxicity has usually involved studies in two or more species of animals that are exposed by the routes and in the concentrations most appropriate for the toxic agent for periods ranging from several months to several years. Such

74

studies are expensive and time-consuming, but there is presently no substitute technique that is adequate for assessing long-term human health hazards. The degree of confidence with which such hazards may be estimated depends on the quality of the toxicological data; therefore, considerable care must be taken in the design, execution, and interpretation of such studies.

It is axiomatic that chronic toxicity studies are performed only after tests for acute and subchronic toxicity have been conducted. Usually the specific tests for toxicity, such as organ toxicity tests, will also have been completed before the chronic toxicity study is initiated. These subchronic studies are, in fact, quite likely to have identified most of the major types of toxicity that will be encountered in the chronic toxicity study except for carcinogenicity and cumulative toxic effects. Acute and subchronic toxicity studies cannot be substituted for the chronic toxicity study, as the acute and chronic toxic effects of chemicals differ. In addition, short-term studies may fail to predict toxic effects that are related to the aging process. However, these studies are of critical importance for the proper planning of the chronic study. The objective of the chronic study is not to confirm positive findings from the subchronic studies. It should provide dosage information on the toxicity shown in the short-term studies so that toxicity can be avoided, i.e., to establish a no-observed-effect dosage.

Another major objective of the chronic test is to evaluate the potential tumorigenicity of the test compound. The only conclusive data that implicates a compound as a tumorigenic agent are obtained in the *in vivo* chronic test. In the near future additional work may support an increased confidence in the value of short *in vitro* tests for carcinogenicity (cf. the *in vitro* Ames-type test using microsomal enzyme metabolic systems), at least when negative test results are obtained.

A compound must have considerable economic importance or at least be of academic interest if it reaches the stage where it is considered for chronic studies. Once the decision has been made to undertake a chronic toxicity study, every effort must be made to ensure that the test will produce data that are valid, relevant, and applicable to the experimental or clinical situation and that all of the available information has been extracted from the study. To accomplish these aims, professional judgment must be exercised throughout the study, particularly in the critical areas of dose-level selection, clinical evaluation of the test animals, and interpretation of the results. The elements of good laboratory practice (proper record-keeping, data verification, protocol adherence, and justification of deviations from protocol) should be employed throughout such tests.

No single set of toxicity tests protocols will be adequate in every experiment. The recommendations in the subsequent sections of this report are minimal guidelines for the toxicological evaluation of a chemical agent.

## DESIGN OF TEST

### THE TEST AGENT AND ITS PREPARATION

Household substances are comprised of a wide variety of liquid, solid, and aerosol products. In evaluating the safety of these substances, careful attention must be given to the physical form of the test material. Specialized facilities are required for the safety evaluation of gases and aerosols (see Chapter 4). In certain instances, dermal toxicity tests may be required (see Chapter 3).

The purity and chemical composition of the test substance should be rigorously evaluated prior to undertaking toxicity tests. As much information as possible should be obtained on the chemical nature of ingredients of mixtures, including their stability, the nature of chemical impurities, the chemical form of the vehicle or diluent, and the physical properties of the test substance at room temperature. To assist in the interpretation of the results of toxicity studies, only one lot of the test substance should be used in toxicity tests; however, data should be available on interlot variation.

Liquids may be administered by gavage or admixed in the drinking water, if they are soluble. The most convenient method of administration in chronic toxicity testing is via the diet. Both liquids and finely ground solids may be incorporated into animal rations. The stability of the test substance in the diet must be determined. Its toxicity may be altered by interaction with dietary constituents, or principal toxic agents may be lost due to their vapor pressure.

### DIET

The diet fed to the test animals should meet all of their nutritional requirements[16] and promote longevity. It should be free of toxic impurities that could influence the outcome of the toxicity test. Batches of the diet should be analyzed for pesticides (chlorinated hydrocarbons, etc.), mycotoxins (aflatoxins, ochratoxins, etc.), and industrial contaminants such as PCB's, lead, and mercury.

Commercially available diets of recognized quality are suitable for most toxicity studies, but occasionally, when the nutrient composition requires alteration to achieve nutritional balance among test groups, semipurified diets may be used.[15,18] Fresh feed should be provided as often as necessary, but at least weekly. Rodents should be fed *ad libitum*. Nonrodents may be given fresh feed daily. Periodically, the diet should be analyzed for nutrient content, as major alterations in diet composition may affect the nature of toxic responses.[2,10]

## SELECTION OF SPECIES AND STRAIN

The species of animals used in chronic toxicity testing will depend, to a large degree, on the test objectives. Metabolic and physiological considerations must be included in the selection process. If the metabolism of the test compound is known in man, the metabolism of the species selected should respond similarly. For example, the rat or mouse are of limited value for studying the neurotoxicity of methylmercury compounds, because rodents, unlike humans, rapidly metabolize these compounds to a less toxic inorganic form.[17] Cats and nonhuman primates metabolize these compounds similarly to humans. They are, therefore, more appropriate test species.[7,11] The use of dogs, cats, and nonhuman primates is sometimes indicated when studying the neurotoxic properties of chemicals, as neurological testing procedures are well established in these species.[7,13,14]

In carcinogenicity assays, because of the large number of animals needed and the requirement to conduct studies for most of the animals' lives, choice is restricted to rats, mice, or hamsters. Certain strains of these species have become widely accepted as test animals in carcinogencity bioassay because a great deal is known about their spontaneous tumor incidence, sensitivity to tumor induction, availability, genetic stability, hardiness, and longevity.[20]

When there is little information on the metabolism or toxicity of the test substance in humans, the results of subchronic toxicity, metabolic, and pharmacodynamic studies will aid considerably in the selection of test species. In general, the species and strain showing the greatest sensitivity in subchronic studies should be selected for chronic toxicity studies provided that it does not react atypically to the compound due to metabolic peculiarities.

## NUMBER OF ANIMALS

In chronic toxicity tests involving rodents, particularly in cancer bioassay procedures, it has become accepted practice to use 50 animals of each sex per dose level. Fewer animals per group may be used if the number of dose levels is increased, but Loomis[12] has recommended a minimum of 20 rodents of each sex per group. Range-finding and subchronic studies will provide guidance in the number of animals needed in the chronic toxicity test.[4] The number will also depend on the degree of statistical confidence desired in the toxicity appraisal. When using dogs, cats, or nonhuman primates, each group should consist of a minimum of four animals of each sex. If it is anticipated that interim sacrifices are required, additional animals will be needed. Care must be taken to ensure proper randomization and distribution of littermates in both control and experimental groups.

CONTROL ANIMALS

The quality of data obtained from the test and the statistical evaluation of the results rely heavily on having adequate control data from concurrent controls that were obtained from the same source. Although historical control data may be a valuable source for information on the incidence of neoplastic lesions,[19] disease patterns, or other peculiarities of the specific strain, such data are not considered adequate as control data in toxicity tests.

The control group should contain at least as many animals of each sex as each of the test groups. Some authors[12] recommend that it contain twice as many. Except for treatment with the test substance, the control animals are treated identically to the test animals. All measurements should be conducted on both the treated animals and on the controls. All lesions or other phenomena occurring in the control animals must be carefully noted, as spontaneous disease processes may influence the toxicity of the test substance. In any type of toxicity study, the treated groups should not inadvertently expose the control groups, laboratory workers, or animal caretakers to toxic levels of the test agent. Such laboratory safety considerations are particularly important in chronic toxicity testing. There may also be a need for "positive" controls in order to establish the susceptibility of the test species or strain to the specific toxic effects of the test agent. Such "positive" controls may be essential in detecting borderline effects and minimal enhancement of normal pathological or age-related conditions.


DOSE SELECTION

Doses for chronic toxicity tests may be selected on the basis of results of subchronic studies; however, such an approach is somewhat empirical. It is not uncommon in chronic toxicity tests to find that the top dose group suffers unexpected toxicity during the first year of the study. This is particularly true in the study of such compounds as the halogenated aromatics and some of the alkyl metallics that have slow rates of elimination and tend to accumulate in the tissues. For this reason, it may be helpful to undertake pharmacodynamic studies, including rates of absorption, metabolism, and excretion. These may assist in establishing the behavior of the test substance in the body. Studies of this nature will provide information on the degree to which the test substance may accumulate in various body compartments and produce unexpected toxicity. Particular attention should be given to evidence of dose-dependent detoxification, since metabolic overloading may be produced at high dose levels. Such information is necessary in the interpretation of the toxicity data.

In chronic toxicity testing, the establishment of a no-observed-effect level is usually an objective. To accomplish this a minimum of three dose levels is required. The upper dose level should produce some signs of toxicity but should not greatly alter normal physiological function. The lowest dose level would not be expected to produce evidence of toxicity. When selecting appropriate doses, consideration also should be given to the anticipated level of human exposure and the margin of safety that might be used to evaluate the results of the chronic toxicity test.

DURATION OF STUDY

A basic principle in chronic toxicity testing is that the test animals be exposed to the test substance for a large portion of their life span. This approach, though desirable, is often not attainable in practice, particularly if tests are conducted in long-lived species.

In cancer bioassays with rodents, it is generally agreed that the experiment should start with weanlings and continue for a minimum of 2 yr. When exposure of pregnant women is possible, it should commence *in utero* and continue with the $F_1$ generation for lifetime. In this approach, groups of weanlings are exposed until they reach sexual maturity. They are then bred within dose groups. Following weaning, the offspring are exposed to their parents' diet for their entire lifespan.[6,8] In practice, it may be necessary to sacrifice the remaining animals in the higher-dosage-level groups prior to the end of the study to ensure an adequate number of animals for the pathology studies. Although the point at which the survivors in any group are sacrificed depends on the initial size of the group and mortality rates, most chronic-toxicity-test protocols recommend sacrifice of the remaining animals when their number reaches 20 percent. Excessive mortality in all of the treated groups usually indicates faulty judgment in dose selection or a concurrent disease problem. With nonrodent species, such as dogs or nonhuman primates, lifetime exposures are not feasible. Most studies in these species are terminated after 1 to 2 yr. Terminating nonrodent studies after 1 or 2 yr is strictly an empirical process. Carefully conducted pharmacodynamic studies will assist in establishing when to terminate the study, since data on steady-state characteristics of blood levels may be obtained. Treatment that is continued for a substantial period after the attainment of steady state without any noticeable change in toxic effects will usually provide increased assurance for the selection of sacrifice times.

## TEST PROCEDURE

ROUTE OF ADMINISTRATION

In chronic toxicity tests, the route of administration of the test substance should be similar to the anticipated route of administration in humans. If that route is oral, the test material may be added to the diet or drinking water, or it may be administered by gavage. An advantage of gavage is that dose levels may be quantitated readily. This may be important in defining a no-ob-served-effect level for a substance having a steep dose-response or in instances where a tight dose range is used. Gavage also provides increased control over the handling of hazardous substances.[20] Because it is a tedious technique, many investigators prefer the diet, which is the most convenient means of administration. The test material must be uniformly distributed in the diet and the particles of solids must be sufficiently small so that the animals will not reject them by selection.

In rodent studies, the diet may be administered in two ways: first, by addition of the compound as a fraction of the total diet, or second, by adding a sufficient quantity of the chemical to the diet to achieve predetermined dose levels (in milligrams/kilograms body weight/day). In the latter case, the dietary concentration must be adjusted weekly or biweekly to maintain a constant dose level, since food consumption per unit of body weight decreases as the animal gets older. If the concentration were held constant from weaning to maturity, the actual dose received would be reduced by approximately 2.5 times over the dosing period. This may have profound effects on the severity of the toxic response and may, under some circumstances, be mistaken for tolerance.

In dog studies, administration in the diet is an acceptable route; however, capsule administration may be necessary for unpalatable compounds. The problems encountered in administration via the drinking water are similar to those encountered in diet administration. An added factor, solubility of the test substance, must be considered.

## EVALUATION

### BODY WEIGHT AND FOOD CONSUMPTION

Tests with most rodent species (rats, mice, hamsters) are usually started soon after the animals are weaned. For the first 3 to 6 mo of the study, the animals grow rapidly. Body weights and growth are important measurements of adverse effects. The weights are usually measured weekly during this growth period and monthly thereafter. The frequency should be increased when there are large numbers of tumors or an apparent deterioration in the animals' health. Ideally, weights should be recorded for individual animals. The same examinations and procedures should be used for all test animals, including controls. Larger animals such as dogs and monkeys usually are weighed weekly throughout their lifetimes as an index of growth.

Measurement of food consumption, while of limited value in monitoring a study, nevertheless is useful in determining the dose administered in feed and the effects on food consumption. An alternative to continuous measurement is to measure a representative sampling of each test group for 1 wk each month.

Food efficiency and/or food utilization can be calculated from the amount of intake and growth rate.

### MORTALITY AND REACTIONS

Viability, general physical condition, and adverse behavioral changes of every animal should be checked once each morning and late afternoon for 7 days each week. Animals in poor health with life-threatening conditions should be isolated. Those whose condition makes survival for another 24 h unlikely should be immediately sacrificed and necropsied. Rapid necropsy is particularly desirable in the later stages of the study, so that tissues can be saved for histological examination.

### CLINICAL AND LABORATORY EXAMINATIONS

Astute clinical observations can alert the investigator to the early onset of an infectious disease or degeneration of health due to the test compound. As each animal in a chronic study represents a great investment in time and money, all losses, whether due to disease, unwanted toxicity, autolysis, or cannibalism, must be avoided. The cost of careful and frequent clinical examinations is warranted. Not only can the examinations reduce animal losses, but also they can prove useful for evaluating the test or its results.

Every animal should be carefully examined at least once a week by competent laboratory animal technicians. In addition to an examination for abnormalities of hair coat, eyes, mouth, teeth, nose, and ears, both urine and feces should be checked for discoloration and consistency. The animals should also be palpated for body masses and observed for neurological conditions.

Special clinical examinations, such as electrocardiograms, electroencephalograms, electromyograms, electroretinograms and other ophthalmoscopic examinations, routine X rays, and checks of respiratory rate, respiratory function (particularly in inhalation studies), and neurological function, are usually conducted only on large laboratory animals.

Clinical chemistry tests should be judiciously selected. They may be based on toxicity signs that were manifested during preliminary or short-term toxicity tests, or upon the type of compound being studied. For example, certain organophosphate and carbamate compounds inhibit cholinesterase. In a study with these types of compounds, the activity of cholinesterase in plasma, erythrocytes, and brain should be measured as an index of effects.

There is a battery of possible tests, including organ function tests, hematology tests, and measurement of various blood chemicals.[3,5] Routine urinalyses are of doubtful usefulness.

Many of these tests are now automated and can be performed using microsamples. The sampling procedures should not impair the animal's health. The clinical chemistry determinations should be applicable to humans and be made as necessary or indicated by the health status of the animals. A rigid sampling is impractical and excessively costly.

Organ function tests are most commonly performed on liver and kidneys, the organs most often affected in chronic toxicity tests. All technical personnel involved in conducting these studies should be properly trained and experienced in the techniques. The procedures, data verification, and analysis of results should meet the requirements of good laboratory practice. The tests of organ function can be made on larger animals, but are not usually recommended for rodents. These tests include those for liver function (with BSP), kidney function (with PSP) and thyroid function (with serum iodine, PBI, $T_3$, and $T_4$). The selection of these tests should be left to the discretion of the investigative teams.

## PATHOLOGY EXAMINATIONS

All animals—including those moribund or dying during the study, as well as those at terminal sacrifice—should be carefully necropsied. Selected organs should be closely examined by trained technicians under the supervision of competent animal pathologists. Certain major organs may be weighed as an indication of effects of the compound.[9]

The organs and supporting structures should be fixed in preservatives for histological preparation. The large number of tissues (about 30) from every animal of all test groups as desired by USNCI[20] creates an overwhelming pathology workload. Abrams et al.[1] suggest that pathology examination of 18 different tissues is ample.

As a minimum routine procedure, all major tissues and gross lesions of all high-dose and control animals should be examined microscopically. Grossly altered tissues from animals in other groups should also be included for microscopic examination. Based on the results, investigators can decide whether to examine the remaining tissues from the low-dose groups.

Interim sacrifices are of use in the study of pathogenesis or toxic reactions. They may also yield valuable clues as to the organs that should be more thoroughly examined or to the specific clinical chemistry/organ function tests that should be conducted. Extra animals should be included for this purpose to assure that the number of animals available at the end of the study is statistically sufficient for assessing carcinogenic effects.

## EVALUATION OF DATA

The principles involved in the design and interpretation of chronic toxicity studies are concerned with the detection of a chemical's influence on any function that is associated with the development, maturation, and aging of the test animal. The quality of the data base will determine the interpretation of the results. The principles of good experimental toxicological practice must be incorporated in the protocol. These are:

• The incorporation of concurrent negative controls. It is not acceptable to rely on data from control animals used in prior studies. The controls should be treated identically to the test animals, with the exception of omission of the test chemical.

• A minimum of at least three dose levels should be used. The highest of these should approximate the maximal tolerated dose. During the experiment, the doses should be adjusted to take into account changes in the weight of the animals. Since it is desirable to estimate a "maximal-no-observed-effect" dose and since extrapolation outside the parameters of the experiment is likely to be accompanied by severe inaccuracies, the lowest dose used should bear some relation to the anticipated level of exposure to the compound.

• The chemical involved in the test should be specifically identified including all measurable impurities so that approximately 100 percent of the compound is accounted for. In the case of chemically stable forms of test compounds, it is desirable to conduct the entire chronic test from a single batch of the test chemical.

Since the chronic toxicity test is frequently designed to evaluate the tumorigenic potential of the test compound, the investigator should avoid selecting species that normally have a high incidence of tumors unless this condition is of specific value to the study. The metabolism of the species selected for chronic tests should be as similar as possible to humans for the test compound. The benefits of organ function tests at specified intervals during the chronic test is questionable. Such tests are generally unable to detect accurately the minimal toxicity in such organs as the liver or kidney. Extra animals should be added to each group. They can be sacrificed for complete gross and histopathological examination. This would ensure complete diagnoses for intercurrent illness or unanticipated toxicity. Repeated expert observation and physical examination of the animals, plus periodic body weight measurements, are essential. All animals (including those that may expire during the study) should be thoroughly autopsied. All grossly observed lesions, together with examples of the associated organs, should be examined histologically. All animals that started the test should be clearly accounted for in the final report.

The most valid results of a chronic toxicity test are obtained when a dose-response relationship for any form of observed toxicity can be established from the data. The positive identification of a carcinogenic agent is obtainable in some cases, but an unqualified negative answer is never possible. The establishment of a dose with no observed effect is possible only in a statistical sense, i.e., a statistically derived value that is based on specific probabilities. For most experiments, a $< 5$ percent probability that the figure is in error is acceptable. The only way to decrease the probability of error is to increase the number of animals in each test group. The number required to attain this very high level of confidence could easily become economically prohibitive. Investigators should be aware of the limitations associated with the various statistical procedures that can be used.

A guarantee that a given chemical will not produce untoward effects when exposure is over virtually a lifetime is unattainable. It is then necessary to establish some reasonable level of risk. An acceptable level depends on the type of toxicity, the reversibility or irreversibility of its effects, the economic factors associated with the compound's use, and most important on the number of subjects that could be exposed and the patterns of exposure (extent, type, etc.). When toxicity is irreversible and the compound could be available to the entire human race, the establishment of an acceptable level of risk versus benefit is a complex and difficult task and becomes a matter for a collective sociopolitical judgment.

## REFERENCES

1. Abrams, W. B., G. Zbinden, and R. Bagdon. 1965. Investigative methods in clinical toxicology. J. New Drugs 5:199-207.
2. Arcos, J. C., M. F. Argus, and G. Wolf. 1968. Chemical Induction of Cancer, vol. 1. New York, Academic Press. p. 372.
3. Balazs, T. 1975. Toxic effects of chemicals in the liver. FDA By-Lines 5:291-303.
4. Benitz, K.-F. 1970. Measurement of chronic toxicity. *In*: Paget, G. E., ed. Methods in Toxicology. Oxford, Blackwell Scientific Publications. pp. 82-131.
5. Bergmeyer, H. U. 1965. Methods of Enzymatic Analysis. New York, Academic Press.
6. Canada, Health and Welfare Department. 1973. The Testing of Chemicals for Carcinogenicity, Mutagenicity and Teratogenicity. September.
7. Charbonneau, S. M., I. C. Munro, E. A. Nera, R. F. Willes, T. Kuiper-Goodman, F. Iverson, C. A. Moodie, D. R. Stoltz, F. A. J. Armstrong, J. F. Uthe, and H. C. Grice. 1974. Subacute toxicity of methylmercury in the adult cat. Toxicol. Appl. Pharmacol. 27:569-581.
8. Epstein, S. S. 1969. A "catch-all" toxicological screen. Experientia 25:617.
9. Feron, V. J., A. P. de Groot, M. T. Spanjers, and H. P. Til. 1973. An evaluation of the criterion "organ weight" under conditions of growth retardation. Food Cosmet. Toxicol. 11:85-94.
10. Friedman, L. 1966. Nutritional status and biological response. Fed. Proc. Fed. Am. Soc. Exp. Biol. 25:137-144.
11. Ikeda, Y., M. Tobe, K. Kobayashi, S. Suzuki, Y. Kawasaki, and H. Yonemaru. 1973.

Long-term toxicity study of methylmercuric chloride in monkeys )first report). Toxicology 1:361-375.

12. Loomis, T. A. 1974. Essentials of Toxicology, 2d ed. Philadelphia, Lea & Febiger.
13. McGrath, J. T. 1960. Neurological Examination of the Dog with Clinicopathological Observations, 2d ed. Philadelphia, Lea & Febiger.
14. Mowbray, J. B., and T. E. Cadell. 1962. Early behavior patterns in rhesus monkeys. J. Comp. Physiol. Psychol. 55:350-357.
15. Munro, I. C., C. A. Moodie, D. Krewski, and H. C. Grice. 1974. Carcinogenicity study of commercial saccharin in the rat. Toxicol. Appl. Pharmacol. 32:513-526.
16. National Academy of Sciences-National Research Council. 1972. Committee on Animal Nutrition, Subcommittee on Laboratory Animal Nutrition. Nutrient Requirements of Laboratory Animals, 2d rev. ed. Nutrient Requirements of Domestic Animals, No. 10. Washington, D.C.
17. National Institute of Public Health. 1971. Methylmercury in fish: A toxicologic-epidemiologic evaluation of risks. Report of an expert group. Nord. Hyg. Tidskr. 4 (Suppl.).
18. Newberne, P. M., A. E. Rogers, and G. N. Wogan. 1968. Hepatorenal lesions in rats fed a low lipotrope diet and exposed to aflatoxin. J. Nutr. 94:331-343.
19. Sher, S. P. 1972. Mammary tumors in control rats: Literature tabulation. Toxicol. Appl. Pharmacol. 22:562-588.
20. U.S. National Cancer Institute, Division of Cancer Cause and Prevention. 1976. Guidelines for Carcinogen Bioassay in Small Rodents, by J. M. Sontag, N. P. Page, and U. Saffiotti. Washington, D.C., Government Printing Office. NCI Carcinogenesis Technical Report Series No. 1. DHEW Publication No. (NIH) 76-801.

# $6$ Mutagenicity Tests

Genetic disease in humans shares with infectious disease the dual characteristics of transmission from one individual to another and frequent cryptic transmission in the carrier state. It differs fundamentally, however, not only in patterns of transmission and underlying disease mechanism, but also in that it cannot be cured and it is cumulative in the event of increased mutation rates or decreased selection pressures.

The severity of genetic disease ranges from the subclinical to the lethal. As much as 10 percent of clinically recognized human disease appears to exhibit a strong genetic component.[40] However, this may be only a fraction of the total human genetic disease burden. Studies of lower organisms indicate that the typical deleterious mutation is only mildly debilitating, even when homozygous. While such mutations in humans would escape clinical detection, they would nevertheless contribute to the average background of ill health, e.g., by increasing susceptibility to nongenetic disease. The total mutation rate in higher animals is believed to be on the order of one new deleterious mutation per diploid individual,[29] to which must be added those mutations persisting from previous generations.

There is no known way of estimating the contribution of mutagenic chemicals to genetic disease in humans. However, legitimate concern that certain chemicals may threaten the integrity of the human genome, and thus the health of future generations, is predicated both on sound theoretical reasoning and on inescapable implications derived from a large body of experimental data.

In addition to sexually transmissible germ cell mutations, body cell mutations are also of concern. A striking correlation exists between chemical mutagenicity and carcinogenicity, which, taken together with large geographical variations in cancer incidence, strongly indicates that environmental facts are related to the cause of most human cancer.[31] In addition, there have been recent hints that other types of human disease (such as arteriosclerosis) are traceable to individual aberrant cells. They may, therefore, have originated by mutation.[5]

Fundamental aspects of mutagenesis have been described by Drake,[13] Auerbach and Kilbey,[4] Auerbach,[3] and Drake and Baltz.[15] General discussions of genetic toxicology are also available.[14,21,39,40] There is also a computerized bibliographical service that can supply information about many specific agents.*

## TEST OBJECTIVES

The primary objective of mutagen testing is to determine whether a chemical has the potential to cause sexually transmissible genetic damage in humans. However, direct methods for assessing mutagenicity in humans do not exist, nor should humans ever be deliberately employed as a mutagen test system. Animal model systems, both mammalian and nonmammalian, together with microbial systems, have therefore been used as approximations to human susceptibility.

The second objective of mutagen testing is to estimate quantitatively the human response to chemicals already identified as mutagens. Many compounds, including chemicals already in widespread use and those whose application is proposed, produce substantial benefits. Decisions concerning their use must therefore be based on risk/benefit comparisons, for which the genetic risks must be quantified.

## DETECTION OF MUTAGENS

There are no practical procedures for assessing the induction of heritable mutations in humans. It is therefore necessary to identify the subhuman test systems that, when properly designed and executed, can produce statistically significant positive results implicating an agent as a potential mutagen in humans.

In the recommended tests (listed in Table 1 and described below), three categories of genetic damage are recognized: chromosome mutations, point mutations, and primary DNA damage. In general, an agent that produces a

---

* The Environmental Mutagen Information Center (EMIC), Biology Division, Oak Ridge National Laboratory, P. O. Box Y, Oak Ridge, TN 37830.

TABLE 1    Recommended Tests for Detecting Mutagens

| Class of Damage Detected | In Vivo Mammalian Tests | Ancillary Tests |
|---|---|---|
| Chromosome mutations | Heritable translocations test Cytogenetic tests<br><br>Dominant lethal test | *Drosophila* test *In vitro* mammalian cytogenetic tests |
| Point mutations | Specific locus test | *Drosophila* recessive lethal test *Salmonella* reversion test *In vitro* mammalian specific locus tests |
| Primary DNA damage | Unscheduled DNA synthesis | *In vitro* mammalian unscheduled DNA synthesis Bacterial repair tests Yeast mitotic recombination tests |

positive result in any of the four *in vivo* mammalian mutational tests should be considered as potentially mutagenic in humans unless there are compelling reasons to believe the contrary.

Since detection of some mutagens in the only available *in vivo* mammalian point mutation test requires large numbers of animals, its applicability is limited. An acceptable alternative is a positive result in any two of the three ancillary point mutation tests and evidence that the compound or its active metabolite reaches the germinal tissue.

While not sufficient to identify potential mutagenicity in humans, a single positive result obtained outside *in vivo* mammalian mutation tests should be regarded as an indication of a need for further investigation.

Although nonmutagenicity in humans cannot be proved, negative results in at least three of the five tests for chromosome mutation and in at least two of the four tests for point mutation constitute scientific evidence for a moderate confidence of nonmutagenicity.


## EVOLUTION OF TEST SYSTEMS AND CRITERIA

Because mutagen testing is a young science, frequent technological improvements are to be expected. Certain tests, which appeared very promising only a few years ago, have already been superceded. The potential user should therefore be aware of the continuing advances in methodology.*

* Consult the Environmental Mutagenesis Branch, National Institute of Environmental Health Sciences, P. O. Box 12233, Research Triangle Park, NC 27709.

Operational definitions of mutagens in humans will necessarily undergo parallel changes. Since changes in both mutagen testing procedures and operational definitions of human mutagens may occur more rapidly than will revisions of this document, this chapter should be revised at least biannually and should, where appropriate, be updated by published supplements.*

## PRINCIPLES OF MUTAGEN TESTING

Mutagen tests must fulfill certain requirements if they are to provide information suitable for the protection of humans. No single extant test meets each of these requirements; therefore, a combination of tests must usually be employed, as exemplified above.

The full spectrum of molecular classes of mutation must be detectable. These include the loss or gain of entire chromosomes; mutations arising from chromosome breaks (or equivalent events), namely deletions, duplications, and rearrangements; and point mutations. The last consist of chromosome mutations that are small enough to affect only a single gene, of additions or deletions of one or a few base pairs, and of base pair substitutions. Criteria for reliably detecting all types of point mutations are notably lacking in the *in vivo* mammalian test systems.

Many nonmutagenic chemicals become mutagenic as a result of metabolic processing. Conversely, some mutagens may be so efficiently inactivated through metabolic action that they become innocuous. Thus, an understanding of the corporeal pharmacology of environmental chemicals is crucial to mutagen testing. A suitable capacity for metabolic activation must be incorporated into any test system other than the intact animal. Two methods are currently available. The first involves the direct incorporation of enzymatically competent mammalian tissue extracts into microbial tests (including cultured mammalian cells). The second involves administering the agent to an animal and then obtaining animal extracts (such as urine or blood) for subsequent analysis in a microbial test. Metabolic activation systems are also under continual development. Improvements are to be expected on a regular basis for a number of years.

The pharmacological importance of such factors as routes of administration should not be underestimated. For example, some intestinal organisms contribute to the mutagenic activation of certain chemicals; therefore, it is important that the routes of exposure be appropriate.

Finally, test systems must display both sensitivity, detecting as broad a spectrum of chemical classes as possible, and accuracy, including reproducibility.

* To determine whether supplements are available, consult the Advisory Center on Toxicology, National Academy of Sciences, Washington, DC 20418.

TEST DEPLOYMENT

The fundamental criteria for defining human mutagenicity or nonmutagenicity are described above. Additional criteria may be required when deciding how and when to test chemicals. These include current and/or anticipated patterns of use and human exposure, stage of product development, number of substances to be tested, available testing resources, relevant legislation, and regulatory status. The available test systems can often be considered as building blocks to be assembled according to specific needs.

Single organisms can sometimes be used to detect both point and chromosomal mutations. Where possible, tests should be performed simultaneously on the same population, not only to decrease effort and expense, but, more importantly, to build a comparative data base with great potential use.

If the chemicals to be tested are structurally related to known mutagens, the battery of tests selected should include those capable of detecting that class of mutagens.

When more chemicals are to be screened than can be put through a definitive battery of tests, a prescreen or tier approach may be used.[6,16] A prescreen can rapidly identify substances that are genetically active and should therefore either be withdrawn from further development or be assigned high priority for definitive testing. Microbial systems are the most suitable for screens of this type except for certain classes of mutagens such as metals. Unscheduled DNA synthesis may also be an appropriate prescreen system.

## TEST PROCEDURES

### CHROMOSOME MUTATIONS

*Heritable Translocation Test*   In contrast to the other *in vivo* tests for chromosomal mutations, the heritable translocation test measures heritable damage. In this procedure parental males are treated and their male progeny collected. The progeny are mated to determine semisterility and sterility. Semisterile or sterile animals are analyzed cytogenetically to confirm the apparent translocation heterozygosity. A disadvantage is the requirement for a relatively large number of animals to diagnose efficiently any significant differences between treated and control populations. Generoso *et al.*[17] and Léonard[24] discuss the technique and its utility for routine screening of chemical mutagens.

*In Vivo Cytogenetics Tests*   The recognition that mutagenicity should be investigated in treated animals to assess human hazard has led to the development of various mammalian tests. Some of the most useful employ both somatic and germinal cells in the rat or mouse. The bone marrow has been the tissue of choice for somatic cells, and the testes for germinal cells. There is diversity of opinion as to the significance of chromosome breaks and gaps (see section below on *in vitro* cytogenetic tests). Cohen and Hirschhorn[11] provide a good overview of procedures for cytogenetic studies in animals. Legator *et al*.[23] discuss a statistical approach to evaluating results utilizing somatic cells.

Human lymphocytes can be examined after exposure to a substance through normal use or accident. These cells can be cultured, induced to divide, and examined for chromosomal abnormalities. Lubs and Samuelson[25] described the variability associated with this procedure. Additionally, one should discount gaps as heritable mutagenic events per se, although they may be totalled to provide an overall picture of the effects produced by a mutagenic substance.

*Dominant Lethal Test*    The dominant lethal test in mice and rats has been the most widely used mutagenicity procedure employing intact animals. Objections to this assay are its relative insensitivity to certain known mutagens and the nonheritable nature of the end point. The most reliable indicator of dominant lethality is a statistically significant increase in the number of early embryonic deaths (dead implantations) when females are mated to mutagen-treated males. In certain instances, the genetic factors causing dominant lethality are chromosomal aberrations and translocations produced in sperm, which preclude development of a fertilized egg much beyond the implantation stage. There is a high correlation between substances producing dominant lethality and those producing translocation heterozygosity. Green and Springer[20] discuss some pharmacological factors that should be considered when performing the dominant lethal test. Green *et al*.[18] propose a more refined approach to dominant lethal testing.

*Drosophila Test*    *Drosophila melanogaster* can be used to detect both numerical and structural chromosomal mutations. Some of the advantages of using *Drosophila* for this purpose are ease of rearing large numbers, short generation time, and well characterized genomes. Also, *Drosophila* can metabolically activate promutagens in a manner similar to animals.[41]

The three major methods for detecting chromosomal mutations in *Drosophila* are the dominant lethal, heritable translocation, and X-Y chromosome loss tests. There is a decided disadvantage, however, in performing the dominant lethal assay in *Drosophila*. Since the unhatched egg is the observed end point, it is not usually feasible to distinguish between effects produced by sperm toxicity or sperm inactivation and those produced by mutant sperm. The X-Y chromosome loss and heritable translocation tests are more relevant because they detect heritable genetic damage, the main objective of mutagenicity testing. Abrahamson and Lewis[1] provide an excellent description of these *Drosophila* tests.

*In Vitro Mammalian Cytogenetic Tests*     Numerous types of cultured mammalian cells have been employed to investigate chemical induction of cytogenetic abnormalities such as gaps, breaks, deletions, and rearrangements. Human lymphocytes can be withdrawn from "unexposed" individuals, induced to grow, subsequently exposed to chemical mutagens, and observed for chromosomal abnormalities. When employing established mammalian cell lines, it should be remembered that specific methods vary among cell lines. Also, it has been reported that P-450-mediated drug metabolizing enzyme systems in established cell lines differ from that of the liver in the intact animal.[30] Since recent reviews in this area are unavailable, a practicing cytogeneticist should be consulted. For a general description of methodology, see Dolimpio *et al.*,[12] Green *et al.*,[19] and Moorhead *et al.*[28]

There has been some controversy regarding the heritability of chromosomal breaks and gaps, particularly whether such effects reliably reveal genetic damage. Since they are generally not transmitted to daughter cells, these effects are considered to be less relevant than are rearrangements. Advocates of *in vitro* cytogenetics state that rearrangements that are not observed in combination with breaks and gaps are usually attributable to faulty techniques, insufficient exposure times, or inadequate sample sizes. The technique is doubtlessly useful as a screen for potential mutagens, although it cannot yield definitive information regarding heritability of the observed aberrations. The relationships between gene and chromosomal mutations in the same cell line have been insufficiently investigated. The development of information of this type could establish the quantitative and qualitative relationships among these effects and could lead eventually to a better risk assessment.

POINT MUTATIONS

*Specific Locus Test*     The specific locus test in mice, as developed by Russell,[32] detects specific gene mutations induced in the germ cells of mice exposed to a mutagen. Male mice of a wild-type strain are treated with the test compound, then mated to females that are homozygous for a number of recessive genes, causing visible changes in phenotypes. Normal offspring are wild type; mutants are phenotypically different and easily identified. The primary disadvantage when evaluating chemical mutagens is the requirement for a large number of animals per dose level and the length of performance time compared to other procedures. However, if mutants are obtained, their genotypes can be confirmed through breeding studies. In this respect, the specific locus test is similar to the heritable translocation test, which uses a combination of animal breeding and cytogenetic analysis to confirm the presumptive genetic end point. Of concern is that the specific type of mutagenic event induced cannot be well determined. Small deletions cannot be distinguished from point mutations, even through breeding tests. This, in turn, reduces confidence that true point mutations are detected. Thus, the mouse-specific locus test would only be used following extensive preliminary studies with a series of other assays. Its primary function would be the estimation of germ cell risk related to exposure of a mammal to a mutagenic substance. The procedures for measuring specific locus mutations in mice have been discussed by Cattenach.[8]

*Drosophila Recessive Lethal Test*    *Drosophila melanogaster*, extensively used in genetic studies, appears well suited to the evaluation of chemicals for mutagenic activity. The X-linked recessive lethal test is one of the most reliable. It is capable of measuring mutagenic effects only a few times the spontaneous background. A large number of genes are screened in this assay, which contributes to its sensitivity and reproducibility. The test is relatively rapid (involving only two generations), and mutation induction is easily detected as a lack of certain male progeny in the second generation. Specific procedures for evaluating chemicals with *Drosophila*, including the X-linked recessive lethal test, have been described by Abrahamson and Lewis.[1]

*Salmonella Reversion Test*    A reverse mutation system, using auxotrophic mutants of *Salmonella typhimurium* blocked at various steps in histidine (*his*) biosynthesis, appears to have great utility in screening for chemicals with mutagenic potential. The mutant strains revert to prototrophy by single base pair substitutions (e.g., strain TA-1535) or by base pair insertions and deletions (e.g., strains TA-1537 and TA-1538). The original set of tester strains has undergone several modifications, which, in general, increase their sensitivity to mutagens. The modifications are deletion of the excision repair system, mutation that promotes the penetration of chemicals into the cells, and incorporation of mutability-promoting R-factors into TA-1538 and TA-1535, resulting in strains TA-98 and TA-100, respectively. These two new strains are effective in detecting at least some mutagens not detected with the three original strains.

For general mutagen screening, the test substance and cells from a specific tester strain are incorporated into a soft overlay agar and plated on a selective, bottom-agar base. The assay can screen for the production of mutagenic metabolites by incorporating a microsome activation system into the overlay just prior to plating on the selective agar base. Discussion of *in vitro* activation systems is included in the general procedures given by Ames *et al.*[2] Although most substances can be tested using this procedure, the bacterial assay is very flexible. It can be used to evaluate many types of substances, including liquids, solids, gases, and also highly toxic substances. The test is rapid, economical, and sensitive, permitting large numbers of chemicals to be screened. The availability of a large data base for this procedure,[26,27] containing results from tests on many classes of chemicals, is extremely valuable when evaluating previously untested substances.

*In Vitro Mammalian Specific Locus Tests*    Several mammalian cell lines with karyotypic stability, high plating efficiency, and short generation times have been employed to detect the induction of specific locus mutation.[9,33,35] These assays offer the advantage over microbial and insect mutation systems that the target cells are mammalian. Two of the most frequently used selective systems involve salvage pathways for purines (mutants defective in hypoxanthine-guanine phosphoribosyl transferase [HGPRT]) and pyrimidine (mutants defective in thymidine kinase [TK]).

The most extensively validated assay employing cultured mammalian cells appears to be the mouse lymphoma line L5178Y (TK+/−). This line is heterozygous at the TK locus and will detect forward mutation from TK+/− to TK−/− (thymidine-kinase-deficient cells). An advantage of the L5178Y test is that it is a forward mutation assay and lacks the potential problems of chemical specificity inherent in all reverse mutation systems. The TK−/− mutant cells are identified by cloning treated populations of TK+/− cells in soft-cloning agar, which contains the thymidine analog 5-bromodeoxyuridine (BUdR). This pyrimidine is toxic to cells having a functional thymidine kinase (TK+/−), but not to thymidine-kinase-defective TK−/− cells. The result is that TK−/− cells form clones in the BUdR-supplemented cloning medium. Although the methodology and preliminary validation of this assay have been completed, the test cannot be considered a routine procedure as can the *Salmonella* or *Drosophila* tests. *In vitro* microsomal activation systems can be included with this test to enhance its utility. Detailed procedures for this assay have been described by Clive and Spector.[10]

### PRIMARY DNA DAMAGE

DNA repair tests do not measure mutation per se, but rather damage to DNA induced by chemical treatment of the indicator cells. Microbial test systems measure this type of damage as cell killing. Both *in vivo* and *in vitro* mammalian test systems measure the damage to DNA, either directly or indirectly as it is being repaired.

*In Vivo Unscheduled DNA Synthesis*   Unscheduled DNA synthesis has recently been detected in germ cells of exposed mice. In this assay, the animals are exposed to the mutagen and ³H-thymidine. Measurement of radioactive uptake in meiotic and postmeiotic germ cells indicates mutagen-DNA interaction. A complete discussion of the rationale and methodology for this procedure has been published by Sega.[34]

*In Vitro Mammalian Unscheduled DNA Synthesis*   An assay employing human diploid WI-38 cells measures unscheduled DNA synthesis (UDS). Following growth in normal medium, the WI-38 cells are blocked in the G phase of the cell cycle by a combination of amino acid depletion and hydroxyurea treatment. The blocked cells are then exposed to the test substance and ³H-thymidine. After treatment, the amount of ³H-thymidine that is incorporated into the nonreplicating DNA is measured by autoradiography or by extraction and scintillation counting of the DNA. The amount of UDS is assumed to be directly related to the extent of damaged DNA produced by chemical treatment. Procedures for this type of assay have been described by Stich *et al.*[37] Although DNA repair is a nonmutagenic end point, there appears to be a good correlation between the ability of a chemical to induce both effects.[38]

*Bacterial Repair Test*   A microbial test system employing bacterial indicator cells has been used extensively. The strains usually employed are *E. coli* W3110 (*polA*+) and P3478 (*polA*−). The latter is deficient in DNA polymerase and unable to carry out excision repair of damaged DNA.[22] The repair test consists of exposing *polA*+ and *polA*− cells to a given concentration of the test material, then measuring the cells that are killed as a result of the exposure. If the substances damage DNA, the *polA*− strain will exhibit enhanced sensitivity to the material compared to the *polA*+ strain. If there is no cell killing or the damage is not related to DNA, sensitivity to the substance will be similar for both bacterial strains. The assay can be conducted as a plate or a suspension test.[36]

*Yeast Mitotic Recombination Tests*   Mitotic crossing over (MCO) and mitotic gene conversion (MGC) can easily be detected in appropriately constructed diploid strains of the yeast *Saccharomyces cerevisiae*. Many chemicals have been screened for genetic activity in strains $D_3$ (MCO), $D_5$ (MCO), and $D_4$ (MGC) of yeast.[43]

MCO is detected by the production of homozygosity in diploid strains that are heterozygous at one or more loci. The MCO events in $D_3$ and $D_5$ are identified by the accumulation of a red or pink pigment that is produced when certain *ade-2* alleles become homozygous.[7] MGC is detected by the ability of cells to form colonies on unsupplemented selective medium.[42]

Although neither MCO or MGC represent mutagenic end points, chemicals that are mutagenic in yeast also produce some type of mitotic recombination, often at concentrations lower than those required to produce mutagenic effects.

Methods for the adaptation of *in vitro* microsome activation systems to yeast assays have been reported by Brusick and Andrews.[7]

The yeast strains $D_3$, $D_4$, and $D_5$ offer certain features not found in other microbial assays: They are diploid eukaryotic strains; they detect genetic damage of a nature not identified in bacteria assays but which may be relevant to diploid cells proliferating in an environment containing genetically active chemicals; and they appear to respond to both mutagenic (base substitution and frameshift classes) and clastogenic chromosome breaking agents. Detailed procedures for the use of these yeast strains have been provided by Zimmermann.[44]

## REFERENCES

1. Abrahamson, S., and E. B. Lewis. 1971. The detection of mutations in *Drosophila melanogaster*. *In*: Hollaender, A., ed. Chemical Mutagens: Principles and Methods for Their Detection, vol. 2. New York, Plenum. pp. 461-487.
2. Ames, B. N., J. McCann, and E. Yamasaki. 1975. Methods for detecting carcinogens and mutagens with the Salmonella/mammalian-microsome mutagenicity test. Mutat. Res. 31:347-364.
3. Auerbach, C. 1976. Mutation Research: Problems, Results and Perspectives. London, Chapman and Hall; distributed in the United States by Halsted Press, New York.
4. Auerbach, C., and B. J. Kilbey. 1971. Mutation in eukaryotes. Annu. Rev. Genet. 5:163-218.
5. Benditt, E. P., and J. M. Benditt. 1973. Evidence for a monoclonal origin of human atherosclerotic plaques. Proc. Natl. Acad. Sci. USA 70:1753-1756.
6. Bridges, B. A. 1973. Some general principles of mutagenicity screening and a possible framework for testing procedures. Environ. Health Perspect. 6:221-227.
7. Brusick, D., and H. Andrews. 1974. Comparison of the genetic activity of dimethylnitrosamine, ethyl methanesulfonate, 2-acetylaminofluorene and ICR-70 in *Saccharomyces cerevisiae* strains $D_3$, $D_4$ and $D_5$ using *in vitro* assays with and without metabolic activation. Mutat. Res. 26:491-500.
8. Cattanach, B. M. 1971. Specific locus mutation in mice. *In*: Hollaender, A., ed. Chemical Mutagens: Principles and Methods for Their Detection, vol. 2. New York, Plenum. pp. 535-539.
9. Chu, E. H. Y. 1971. Induction and analysis of gene mutations in mammalian cells in culture. *In*: Hollaender, A., ed. Chemical Mutagens: Principles and Methods for Their Detection, vol. 2. New York, Plenum. pp. 411-444.
10. Clive, D., and J. F. S. Spector. 1975. Laboratory procedure for assessing specific locus mutations at the TK locus in cultured L5178Y mouse lymphoma cells. Mutat. Res. 31: 17-29.
11. Cohen, M. M., and K. Hirschhorn. 1971. Cytogenetic studies in animals. *In*: Hollaender, A., ed. Chemical Mutagens: Principles and Methods for Their Detection, vol. 2. New York, Plenum. pp. 515-534.

12. Dolimpio, D. A., C. Jacobson, and M. Legator. 1968. Effect of aflatoxin on human leuko-cytes. Proc. Soc. Exp. Biol. Med. 127:559-562.
13. Drake, J. W. 1970. The Molecular Basis of Mutation. San Francisco, Holden-Day.
14. Drake, J. W., *Chairman*. 1975. Environmental mutagenic hazards. Prepared by Committee 17 of the Environmental Mutagen Society. Science 187:503-514.
15. Drake, J. W., and R. H. Baltz. 1976. The biochemistry of mutagenesis. Annu. Rev. Biochem. 45:11-37.
16. Flamm, W. G. 1974. A tier system approach to mutagen testing. Mutat. Res. 26:329-333.
17. Generoso, W. M., W. L. Russell, S. W. Huff, S. K. Stout, and D. G. Gosslee. 1974. Effects of dose on the induction of dominant-lethal mutations and heritable translocations with ethyl methanesulfonate in male mice. Genetics 77:741-752.
18. Green, S., F. M. Moreland, and W. G. Flamm. 1975. A more refined approach to dominant lethal testing. Mutat. Res. 31:340-341. Abstract no. 62.
19. Green, S., K. A. Palmer, and M. S. Legator. 1970. *In vitro* cytogenetic investigation of calcium cyclamate, cyclohexylamine and triflupromazine. Food Cosmet. Toxicol. 8:617-623.
20. Green, S., and J. A. Springer. 1975. Additional statistical evaluation and pharmacological considerations of hycanthone methanesulfonate-induced dominant lethality. J. Toxicol. Environ. Health 1:293-299.
21. Hollaender, A., ed. 1971-1976. Chemical Mutagens: Principles and Methods for Their Detection, vols. 1-4. New York, PLENUM.
22. Kelly, R. B., M. R. Atkinson, J. A. Huberman, and A. Kornberg. 1969. Excision of thymine dimers and other mismatched sequences by DNA polymerase of *Escherichia coli*. Nature 224:495-501.
23. Legator, M. S., K. A. Palmer, and I. D. Adler. 1973. A collaborative study of *in vivo* cyto-genetic analysis. I. Interpretation of slide preparations. Toxicol. Appl. Pharmacol. 24:337-350.
24. Léonard, A. 1973. Observations of meiotic chromosomes of the male mouse as a test of the potential mutagenicity of chemicals in mammals. *In*: Hollaender, A., ed. Chemical Muta-gens: Principles and Methods for Their Detection, vol. 3. New York, Plenum. pp. 21-56.
25. Lubs, H. A., and J. Samuelson. 1967. Chromosome abnormalities in lymphocytes from normal human subjects. A study of 3,720 cells. Cytogenetics 6:402-411.
26. McCann, J., E. Choi, E. Yamasaki, and B. N. Ames. 1975. Detection of carcinogens as mutagens in the *Salmonella*/microsome test: Assay of 300 chemicals. Proc. Natl. Acad. Sci. USA 72:5135-5139.
27. McCann, J., N. E. Spingarn, J. Kobori, and B. N. Ames. 1975. Detection of carcinogens as mutagens: Bacterial tester strains with R factor plasmids. Proc. Natl. Acad. Sci. USA 72:979-983.
28. Moorhead, P. S., P. C. Nowell, W. J. Mellman, D. M. Battips, and D. A. Hungerford. 1960. Chromosome preparations of leukocytes cultured from human peripheral blood. Exp. Cell Res. 20:613-616.
29. Mukai, T., S. I. Chigusa, L. E. Mettler, and J. F. Crow. 1972. Mutation rate and dominance of genes affecting viability in *Drosophila melanogaster*. Genetics 72:335-355.
30. Owens, I. S., and D. W. Nebert. 1974. Aryl hydrocarbon hydroxylase induction in mam-malian liver-derived cell cultures. Stimulation of "cytochrome $P_1450$-associated" enzyme activity by many inducing compounds. Mol. Pharmacol. 11:94-104.
31. Raucher, F. J., Jr., and W. G. Flamm. In press. Introduction to the etiology of cancer. *In*: Holland, J. F., and E. Frei, eds. Cancer Medicine, 2d ed. Philadelphia, Lea & Febiger.
32. Russell, W. L. 1951. X-ray-induced mutations in mice. Cold Spring Harbor Symp. Quant. Biol. 16:327-336.

33. Sato, K., R. S. Slesinski, and J. W. Littlefield. 1972. Chemical mutagenesis at the phosphoribosyltransferase locus in cultured human lymphoblasts. Proc. Natl. Acad. Sci. USA 69:1244-1248.
34. Sega, G. A. 1974. Unscheduled DNA synthesis in the germ cells of male mice exposed *in vivo* to the chemical mutagen ethyl methanesulfonate. Proc. Natl. Acad. Sci. USA 71: 4955-4959.
35. Shapiro, N. I., A. E. Khalizev, E. V. Luss, M. I. Marshak, O. N. Petrova, and N. B. Varshaver. 1972. Mutagenesis in cultured mammalian cells. I. Spontaneous gene mutations in human and Chinese hamster cells. Mutat. Res. 15:203-214.
36. Slater, E. E., M. D. Anderson, and H. S. Rosenkranz. 1971. Rapid detection of mutagens and carcinogens. Cancer Res. 31:970-973.
37. Stich, H. F., R. H. C. San, and Y. Kawazoe. 1971. DNA repair synthesis in mammalian cells exposed to a series of oncogenic and non-oncogenic derivatives of 4-nitroquinoline 1-oxide. Nature 229:416-419.
38. Stoltz, D. R., L. A. Poirier, C. C. Irving, H. F. Stich, J. H. Weisburger, and H. C. Grice. 1974. Evaluation of short-term tests for carcinogenicity. Toxicol. Appl. Pharmacol. 29: 157-180.
39. Sutton, H. E., and M. I. Harris, eds. 1972. Mutagenic Effects of Environmental Contaminants. New York, Academic Press.
40. U.S. Department of Health, Education, and Welfare. 1977. Approaches to the Mutagenic Properties of Chemicals: Risk to Future Generations. Prepared for the DHEW Committee to Coordinate Toxicology and Related Programs by working group of the Subcommittee on Environmental Mutagenesis.
41. Vogel, E. 1975. Some aspects of the detection of potential mutagenic agents in *Drosophila*. Mutat. Res. 29:241-250.
42. Zimmermann, F. K. 1971. Induction of mitotic gene conversion by mutagens. Mutat. Res. 11:327-337.
43. Zimmermann, F. K. 1973. Detection of genetically active chemicals using various yeast systems. *In*: Hollaender, A., ed. Chemical Mutagens: Principles and Methods for Their Detection, vol. 3. New York, Plenum. pp. 209-239.
44. Zimmermann, F. K. 1975. Procedures used in the induction of mitotic recombination and mutation in the yeast *Saccharomyces cerevisiae*. Mutat. Res. 31:71-86.

# 7 Reproduction and Teratogenicity Tests

The objective of teratogenicity testing is the identification of agents acting during embryonic development to produce or alter the incidence of congenital malformations and during the fetal period to produce functional changes in the offspring. Teratogenicity from chemical agents and physical forces is a very real hazard to humans. No single animal test will provide assurances of safety. Because of the many factors involved in chemical-induced teratogenesis, extrapolation of the dose-response relationship from animals to humans is difficult and arbitrary. Chemical-induced teratogenesis is dose-related, but, beyond that, little is really understood concerning the minimal dose of most chemicals that can produce teratogenesis in humans or the extent of the variability in human responses. At present, if any chemical is teratogenic in any animal species at a dosage below apparent maternal toxicity, then the possible hazard of teratogenicity in humans must be fully considered before the chemical is released for public use. Thus, teratogenicity testing in animals can only be regarded as an indication of probability that the test substance will or will not act similarly in humans. Animal testing may also enable identification of teratogens, which are unlikely to be identified by available epidemiological techniques.

Tests to evaluate relevant developmental changes in morphology and functions during perinatal development are desirable. Procedures for recognition of functional deviations in a fetus or neonate are available and referenced, but are not recommended for routine testing unless there is a reason to suspect functional impairment. Teratogenic assessment is presently limited to external, gross visceral, and skeletal examinations. Microscopic examination of viscera can make the screening procedures more effective.

Overall reproductive efficiency can be evaluated through multigeneration studies. A multigeneration reproduction study provides information on fertility and pregnancy in parent and subsequent generations. The effects of a potentially toxic substance could be determined by the reproductive performance through successive generations.

To design suitable protocols for evaluating a substance's potential effects on reproduction, one should consider the various aspects of teratogenicity screening. Screening methods should be improved whenever possible. New methods should be soundly based on new or unapplied interdisciplinary knowledge.

The protocols described in this chapter are examples. Testing protocols should be individualized, based on physical, chemical, and pharmacological properties of the substance to be tested.

## ROUTES OF EXPOSURE

Exposure could occur by inhalation, contact with skin or mucosa, and/or ingestion. The major route of entry during normal use should be investigated. If two or more routes are equally significant, a combination of routes simulating human exposure conditions should be tested. Departure from this concept occurs only when technical or other reasons make it nonfeasible.

Because inhalation is the principal route for aerosols and vapors, teratogenicity testing should be conducted in inhalation chambers. Operation of the chambers, generation and characterization of aerosols and vapors, monitoring of chamber concentrations of test agents, sampling for homogeneous and reproducible distribution of the test materials, regulation of air flow rates, etc., have been described in Chapter 4. For teratogenicity studies, the exposure period is 6 h/day and extends throughout organogenesis. Control animals are maintained under similar experimental conditions. During exposure, the animals are normally unrestrained and individually caged. Position of cages are periodically rotated to equalize any difference in exposure, temperature, and humidity.

When the percutaneous route is chosen, the test agent is applied daily on shaved areas between the shoulders and along the back (25 cm$^2$/rat; 200 cm$^2$/rabbit). The dosages are expressed as milligrams per kilogram of body weight per day. Applications are made evenly over the shaved area by a method designed to deliver precise dosages. When solubility is a limiting factor, the total area for topical application may be varied, or else several applications at the same site may be useful to obtain the desired dose levels. Whether the treated skin is rinsed at a particular time after application or left unrinsed between daily applications will depend on the mode of human usage of the test material. Ingestion from licking is prevented by covering the treated skin with a plastic guard or, if needed, by using restraining devices.[11] During the period of cutaneous applications, the skin is carefully examined every day, and hair growth is controlled by repeated clippings.

If exposure to a given substance is via the digestive tract, it should be dosed orally. The test substance may be administered by intragastric or intraesophageal intubation or by mixing in the diet or drinking water. These three methods might produce slightly different fetal or maternal responses. Selection, therefore, will be based on the best simulation of the human exposure route. Daily food and water consumption records will be required so that dosage can be calculated and palatability of the mixture of test material and food or water can be assured. The dosages will be expressed as milligrams per kilogram of body weight per day.

## DOSE LEVEL, VEHICLE, ANIMAL MODEL, AND ANIMAL ENVIRONMENTS

A substance might produce different effects than those produced by its individual chemical components. When possible, products are tested without changing their ingredients. If a vehicle is administered with the test substance, the control animals are given an equivalent amount of the vehicle. The vehicles used are nontoxic and should not appreciably change the bioavailability and pharmacokinetics of the test agent or alter the physiology and visceral histology of the test animals. If the test substance is administered without a vehicle added, controls will be sham-treated.

At least three dose levels should be selected in a geometric progression. The highest test dose should be the maximum tolerated dose that generally produces about 1 percent lethality. The lowest dose should produce no significant fetal effects. The middle dose is useful for evaluating dose-effect relationship of the observed effects. To estimate accurately the three dosages, a preliminary study at several dosage levels during organogenesis is highly desirable. It may also alert the investigator to the type of effects that might be expected.

At least two species should be used. Although mouse, rat, and rabbit have been selected most frequently, testing is not restricted to these species (see Table 1).

Fetal development is influenced by maternal environments (nutrition, housing, temperature, light, humidity, and overcrowding), genotype of the mother and the fetus, and interaction of these factors. Every effort should be made to keep environmental factors under controlled conditions.[9,10,18]

TABLE 1 Reproductive Events of Mammals, in days[a]

| Species | Sexual Maturity[b] | Estrus Cycle Recurrence | Implantation | Primitive Streak | Duration of Organogenesis | Length of Gestation |
|---|---|---|---|---|---|---|
| Hamster | 42.0-54.0 | 4.0 | 4.5-5.0 | 6.0 | 7.0-14.0 | 16.0-17.0 |
| Mouse | 28.0 | 4.0-5.0 | 4.5-5.0 | 7.0 | 7.5-16.0 | 20.0-21.0 |
| Rat | 46.0-53.0 | 4.0-5.0 | 5.5-6.0 | 8.5 | 9.0-17.0 | 21.0-22.0 |
| Rabbit | 120.0-240.0 | no est. cycle | 7.0 | 6.5 | 7.0-20.0 | 31.0-32.0 |
| Guinea pig | 84.0 | 13.0-20.0 | 6.0 | 10.0 | 11.0-25.0 | 65.0-68.0 |
| Pig | 200.0-210.0 | 19.0-23.0 | 10.0-12.0 | 11.0 | 12.0-34.0 | 110.0-116.0 |
| Sheep | 150.0-300.0 | 16.5 | 10.0 | 13.0 | 14.0-35.0 | 142.0-150.0 |
| Cat | 210.0-245.0 | 14.0 | 13.0-14.0 | 13.0 | 14.0-26.0 | 58.0-71.0 |
| Dog | 270.0-425.0 | 182.5 | 13.0-14.0 | 13.0 | 14.0-30.0 | 57.0-66.0 |
| Rhesus monkey | 1,642.0 | 24.0-38.0 | 9.0 | 18.0 | 20.0-45.0 | 164.0-168.0 |

[a]Compiled from Boyer,[3] Christie,[4] Gruneberg,[8] Nicholas,[12] UFAW,[17] Witschi,[19] and others. Day on which evidence of mating is observed is defined as day 0 of gestation.

[b]Ranges depend on species, nutrition, and other factors.

FETAL EVALUATION

To distinguish between a minor variation and a malformation is difficult. The rate of spontaneous malformations and range in each strain must be determined in each laboratory using the same study procedure as in the testing situation. This is best done, not only by the routine study of control animals in each test, but also by keeping cumulative records of variations observed in all untreated and treated control animals studied by comparable methods. After treatment with a test agent, not only defects that are traditionally recognized as malformations (cleft palate, renal agenesis, club foot, etc.), but also any exceptional, less frequent variations, if the percentage exceeds the range observed in control animals, should usually be regarded as induced malformations.

There is no universally acceptable definition for major or minor malformations. Not all malformations can be extrapolated from laboratory animal studies to humans. Malformations should be ranked according to the degree of deviation from normal and relative significance.

Because developmental derangements may affect biochemistry or functions such as behavior, offspring from the multigeneration study should be observed until sexual maturity for clinical signs and malfunctions. Experience with such animals is insufficient to warrant recommendations for biochemical or functional tests. However, a review of tests for studying variables in postnatal behavioral development has been published. It can be used as a guide for postnatal function testing.[5]

## TERATOLOGY

TEST PROCEDURE

This procedure is designed to determine the effects of substances on embryonic and fetal viability and development. The substances are administered to gravid females upon implantation, then continued through organogenesis. Species with their periods of organogenesis are listed in Table 1.

MATERIAL AND METHODS

Virgin females may be mated naturally by placing them with males. Vaginal smears are taken and females are considered to have mated if spermatozoa and/or a vaginal plug is observed. Day on which evidence of mating is observed is defined as day 0 of gestation. Estrous synchronization and artificial insemination may be used.[1,16,17] Each experiment consists of three treated groups and one control group. Positive control groups will be used as necessary to demonstrate a teratogenic response in the test species. The highest dosage level is the maximum tolerated dosage: The two lower dosages are determined by geometric progression. Twenty mated females are assigned to each group; assignments to groups are made in such a way as to most nearly equalize the day 0 mean group body weights.

## EVALUATION

*Maternal*   Body weights are measured daily during the treatment period and on the day prior to expected delivery. Observation for clinical signs are made daily. Dams showing signs of abortion or premature delivery will be sacrificed on the day such evidence is observed. Reproductive systems and fetuses will be examined for possible abnormalities. These animals will not be included in the final tabulation of data, but will be analyzed separately. Gross necropsy is performed on all animals, including those that die spontaneously or moribund animals that are killed. All dams surviving until the day prior to normal delivery are sacrificed. A thorough postmortem examination is performed, with particular attention paid to the site of administration. If gross changes are observed, histological examination may be conducted.

In these postmortem examinations, several observations should be made and recorded. While examining the uterus, observe and record the number of live fetuses, fetus dying late in gestation (resorbing fetus), and deciduomata (early resorption). In the ovaries, note the number of *corpora lutea* per ovary. All fetuses are tagged individually for identification and then weighed. All fetuses should be examined externally for defects. External sex determination is made when possible.

*Rodents*   After alcohol fixation, gross dissection and examination of viscera are performed on approximately 50 percent of the fetuses of each sex from each litter. Skeletons are examined for anomalies and ossification variations after alizarin-red-staining[6] or other suitable techniques. The remaining fetuses are preserved in Bouin's fluid and examined under a dissecting microscope for neural and visceral defects by serial sectioning[2] or gross dissection.[7,13]

*Nonrodents*   All fetuses are sacrificed. Their sex is determined and internal abnormalities are examined by gross dissection. Skeletal development is evaluated by alizarin-red-staining or by other suitable techniques.

The dead fetuses are weighed and developmental abnormalities are evaluated if autolysis has not advanced. These data are evaluated separately from that of live fetuses.

## REPORT

Data should be compiled in tables presenting maternal mortality, maternal body weights, *corpora lutea*, total implants, deciduoma, fetuses dying late in gestation, live fetuses (number of male and female), fetal weight, and incidence and description of malformation:

$$\text{Pregnancy rate} = \frac{\text{number pregnant}}{\text{number inseminated}} \times 100;$$

$$\text{Implantation efficiency} = \frac{\text{number total implants}}{\text{number corpora lutea}} \times 100; \text{ and}$$

$$\text{Fetal viability} = \frac{\text{number live fetuses}}{\text{number total implants}} \times 100.$$

## STATISTICAL EVALUATION OF DATA

Control and test groups are compared statistically. Anomalies may be compared by chi-square methods[15] or the binomial expansion method. Maternal body weight gains and weight of fetuses may be compared to control by $F$-test and student's $t$-test.[15] When variances differ significantly from control, student's $t$-test may be appropriately modified ($t'$), and Cochran's approximation may be used. Fetal survival and incidence of abnormalities per litter may be compared by a nonparametric, rank-order method.[14] Other statistical methods may be substituted where appropriate.

# REPRODUCTION

## TEST PROCEDURE

The objective of this experiment is to determine the effect on general reproductive performance of treatment commencing at implantation and continuing through the weaning of $F_{2b}$ litters. The preceding teratological study may be included as part of this study.

This experiment is represented schematically in Figure 1. This protocol offers the advantages of predifferentiation exposure of the $F_1$ parental animals without the additional time and costs incurred in a classical two-generation

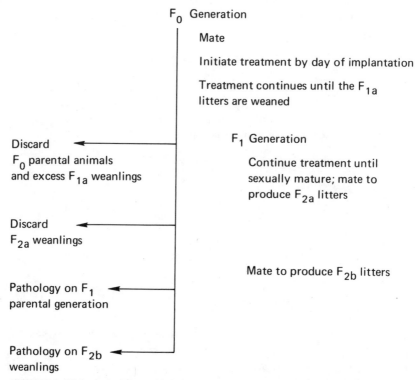

FIGURE 1    Schematic diagram of experiment to determine the effect on general reproductive performance of treatment commencing at implantation and continuing through the weaning of $F_{2b}$ litters.

study. If required, pups may be selected from the $F_{2b}$ litters to produce an $F_3$ generation.

## MATERIALS AND METHODS

The experiments consist of three treatment groups and a control group. Each group consists of 20 sexually mature virgin females mated to a minimum of 10 sexually mature males. The highest dosage is the maximum tolerated dosage. The two lower dose levels are selected by geometric progression. Test materials are administered orally by gavage, mixed in food, or in drinking water (see Chapter 5). Treatment of $F_0$ parental animals may be initiated either on the day of implantation or at the time of pairing. At weaning of the $F_{1a}$ litters, at least 10 males and 20 females are randomly selected from each group to become the $F_1$ parental generation. Selection of both males and females from the same litter should be avoided.

EVALUATION

Body weights and weight gains should be recorded as follows:

- $F_0$ parental females: days 1, 4, 12, 21, and 28 following parturition.
- $F_1$ parental males: weekly from selection until paired for mating.
- $F_1$ parental females: weekly from selection until paired for mating and on days 1, 4, 12, 21, and 28 following parturition of both $F_{2a}$ and $F_{2b}$ litters.
- $F_{1a}$, $F_{2a}$, $F_{2b}$ litters: as litters on days 1, 4, and 12 postparturition and individually at weaning on day 21.

MATING PROCEDURES AND RECORDS

When the $F_1$ parental animals reach sexual maturity (Table 1), each male is randomly mated with two females from the same group. Successful mating is determined by the presence of a copulation plug or blood in the vagina. If a female does not exhibit additional evidence of copulation at the end of a subsequent estrous cycle, she is returned to her original cage. At the end of two estrous cycles, all males within the same group are rotated and exposed to different females in the same group. No more than three males should be paired with any female during a given breeding cycle. The number of observed copulations, the number of estrous cycles required to obtain a mating, and the number of resulting pregnancies should be recorded. These data are used to calculate mating and fertility indices. The $F_{1a}$ litters are weaned at 21 days postpartum, then sacrificed. After an approximately 15-day rest period, the females are mated again. The above procedure is repeated to obtain the $F_{1b}$ litters.

The following indices should be calculated:

$$\text{Mating index} = \frac{\text{number of copulations*}}{\text{number of estrus cycles required}} \times 100$$

$$\text{Fecundity index} = \frac{\text{number of pregnancies}}{\text{number of copulations}} \times 100$$

$$\text{Male fertility index} = \frac{\text{number of males impregnating females}}{\text{number of males exposed to fertile nonpregnant females}} \times 100$$

$$\text{Female fertility index} = \frac{\text{number of females conceiving}}{\text{number of females exposed to fertile males}} \times 100$$

$$\text{Incidence of parturition} = \frac{\text{number of parturitions}}{\text{number of pregnancies}} \times 100$$

* Only one copulation counted per estrus cycle. The rat estrus cycle is 5 days.

## PROGENY PROCEDURES AND RECORDS

All pups ($F_{1a}$, $F_{2a}$, and $F_{2b}$) are examined for physical abnormalities at birth. The numbers of viable, stillborn, and cannibalized members of each litter are recorded. Observations for clinical signs are made daily. The numbers of survivors on days 1, 4, 12, and 21 postparturition are recorded. On the fourth day of lactation, litters with more than 10 pups may be reduced to that number by sacrificing randomly selected individuals. A final examination for physical abnormalities is made. Individual body weights are recorded at weaning on lactation day 21. The following survival indices will be calculated:

$$\text{Live birth index} = \frac{\text{number of viable pups born}}{\text{total number of pups born}} \times 100$$

$$\text{24-h survival index} = \frac{\text{number of pups viable at lactation day 1}}{\text{number of viable pups born}} \times 100$$

$$\text{4-day survival index} = \frac{\text{number of pups viable at lactation day 4}}{\text{number of viable pups born}} \times 100$$

$$\text{12-day survival index} = \frac{\text{number of pups viable at lactation day 12}}{\text{number of pups retained at lactation day 4}} \times 100$$

$$\text{21-day survival index} = \frac{\text{number of pups viable at lactation day 21}}{\text{number of pups retained at lactation day 4}} \times 100$$

## GROSS EXAMINATIONS AND HISTOPATHOLOGY

After the second litter has been weaned (following approximately 33 wk of testing for the rat), 10 male and 10 female $F_1$ parental animals from each group are sacrificed and gross pathological observations are made. Abdominal organs, endocrine glands and gonads, and any other organs that appear abnormal are weighed; organ-to-brain and organ-to-body weight ratios are calculated. A complete set of tissues, including central and peripheral nervous tissue, thoracic and abdominal viscera, and mammary glands, is removed and fixed. Tissues from 5 males and 5 females from both the control and the high-test group are microscopically examined. If histological changes are noted, the target organs of the next-lower-dosage-group animals are also examined. Throughout gross and microscopic examination, particular attention should be paid to the reproductive organs.

Postmortem animals are examined in the same manner, but organ weights are not recorded.

A gross internal examination is made of any pup, $F_{1a}$, $F_{2a}$, or $F_{2b}$, appearing abnormal. In addition, 10 male and 10 female pups, randomly selected from the $F_{2b}$ litters of each test group and the control group, are sacrificed at weaning and subjected to a complete gross examination. Tissues are obtained and preserved as for the $F_1$ parental animals. Histopathological examinations are conducted upon the weanlings of the control and highest-dosage group. If abnormalities are noted, the target organs of the next-lower-dosage-group animals are also examined.

## REPORT

Data are compiled into tables presenting parental body weight, parental organ weight, food consumption (test compound intake), parental mortality, duration of gestation, reproductive data and indices, survival data and indices, progeny body weight, male/female ratio, and histopathological findings.

### STATISTICAL EVALUATION DATA

Control and test groups are compared by statistical methods. Anomalies may be compared by either the chi-square method[15] or the binomial expansion method. Parental body weight gains and weight of progeny may be compared by $F$-test and student's $t$-test.[15] When variances differ appreciably from control, student's $t$-test may be appropriately modified ($t'$), and Cochran's approximation may be used. Survival indices and reproductive indices may be compared by a nonparametric rank order method.[14] Other statistical methods may be substituted where appropriate.

## REFERENCES

1. Adams, C. E. 1961. Artificial insemination in the rabbit. J. Reprod. Fertil. 2:521-522.
2. Barrow, M. V., and W. J. Taylor. 1969. A rapid method for detecting malformations in rat fetuses. J. Morphol. 127:291-305.
3. Boyer, C. C. 1953. Chronology of development for the golden hamster. J. Morphol. 92:1-37.
4. Christie, G. A. 1964. Developmental stages in somite and post-somite rat embryos, based on external appearance, and including some features of the macroscopic development of the oral cavity. J. Morphol. 114:263-286.
5. Coyle, I., M. J. Wayner, and G. Singer. 1976. Behavioral teratogenesis: A critical evaluation. Pharmacol. Biochem. Behav. 4:191-200.
6. Crary, D. D. 1962. Modified benzyl alcohol clearing of alizarin-stained specimens without loss of flexibility. Stain Technol. 37:124-125.
7. Greene, E. C. 1935. The Anatomy of the Rat. New York, Hafner Publishing Co.
8. Gruneberg, H. 1943. The development of some external features in mouse embryos. J. Hered. 34:89-92.

9. National Academy of Sciences-National Research Council, Institute of Laboratory Animal Resources. 1972. Guide for the Care and Use of Laboratory Animals, rev. ed. Washington, D.C., Government Printing Office. DHEW Publication No. (NIH) 74-23.

10. National Academy of Sciences-National Research Council, Institute of Laboratory Animal Resources. 1976. Long-Term Holding of Laboratory Rodents. Washington, D.C.

11. Newmann, E. A. 1963. A new method for restraining rabbits for percutaneous absorption studies. Lab. Anim. Care 13:207-210.

12. Nicholas, J. S. 1949. Experimental methods and rat embryos. In: Farris, E. J., and J. Q. Griffith, Jr., eds. The Rat in Laboratory Investigation, 2d ed. Philadelphia, J. B. Lippincott. pp. 51-67.

13. Rugh, R. 1968. The Mouse: Its Reproduction and Development. Minneapolis, Burgess Publishing Co.

14. Siegel, S. 1956. Nonparametric Statistics for the Behavioral Sciences. New York, McGraw-Hill.

15. Snedecor, G. W., and W. G. Cochran. 1967. Statistical Methods, 6th ed. Ames, Iowa State University Press. pp. 104-219.

16. Sojka, N. J., L. L. Jennings, and C. E. Hamner. 1970. Artificial insemination in the cat (*Felis catus* L.). Lab. Anim. Care 20:198-204.

17. Universities Federation for Animal Welfare (UFAW). 1971. The UFAW Handbook on the Care and Management of Farm Animals. Edinburgh, E. & S. Livingstone.

18. Universities Federation for Animal Welfare. 1976. The UFAW Handbook on the Care and Management of Laboratory Animals, 5th ed. New York, Churchill Livingstone.

19. Witschi, E. 1962. Development of the rat. In: Altman, P. L., and D. S. Dittmer, eds. Growth including Reproduction and Morphological Development. Washington, D.C., Federation of American Societies for Experimental Biology. pp. 304-314.

# 8 Behavioral Toxicity Tests

The many different animal and human behaviors vary widely in their susceptibility to toxic influences. But because the field of "behavioral toxicology" is so young, there has not yet been sufficient systematic experimentation to determine which behaviors are most sensitive to specific toxic agents. To determine that a chemical is free of behavioral effects at any given level of exposure, a great deal of experimentation with many different kinds of behavior is necessary. The fact that one behavioral test shows no effect of a potentially toxic agent does not guarantee that other behaviors will not be affected.[30]

When dealing with a chemical suspected of producing behavioral toxicity, one can start from two possible positions. In one, although acute and chronic toxicity studies have indicated that a potentially toxic agent is safe in many respects at normal exposure levels, an assessment of possible behavioral effects is also desirable. Perhaps, for example, the chemical structure of the compound resembles that of an agent known to have behavioral effects. The question then is: What procedures are appropriate for detecting behavioral effects of chemicals when traditional toxicity testing has given no hint that such effects exist? It seems sensible to turn to rather broad-scale measures that are known to be sensitive to a wide variety of chemicals. Two such procedures are recommended. One is concerned mainly with activity patterns and the other with operant behavior. (These may also be indicated if a behavioral assessment is to take place concurrently with chronic toxicity tests.) In the second situation, signs of behavioral toxicity appear during other

111

toxicological work. For example, a slight ataxia may be seen in animals being tested for the carcinogenic potential of an agent or some signs of defective vision or hearing may be observed. Quantitative confirmation or refutation for a particular finding can be provided by procedures that specifically measure the function in question.

Screening for behavioral toxicity does not differ in principle from screening for other types of toxicity. Methods should be sensitive, quantitative, and reproducible. Other things being equal, a method that is easy to use and inexpensive is preferred to one that is complex and expensive, especially when there is pressure to test numerous and varied commercial products. However, the complex nature of behavior may sometimes preclude the use of simple techniques. More sophisticated methods may be required to discover small and difficult-to-measure changes.

As in other forms of toxicological testing, the probable route of exposure of humans should be reproduced as nearly as possible when studying laboratory animals. Other chapters of this report, particularly those on Inhalation Exposure and Ingestion, should be consulted in this regard. Acute studies should begin with several doses that are high enough to produce obvious effects and then progress to a graded series of smaller doses. Problems of tolerance should be addressed in any of these studies. The resulting acute dose-effect curve can be used to determine appropriate doses for chronic exposure. At least three levels should be used in chronic studies, the minimum effective dose found to affect behavior in acute behavioral studies and two lower doses, with the lowest dose expected to have no observed effects and the intermediate dose at the geometric mean (cf. Chapter 5).

The procedures described below can be used with both rats and mice, two species widely selected for toxicology testing. Behavioral testing methods have been developed for both species. In addition, much is known about the pharmacological sensitivity of these behavioral preparations. Because the procedures can easily be initiated any time after weaning, the age of the animals tested can be selected to correspond to the most sensitive age in humans, either observed or indicated by acute and chronic toxicity data. Behavioral studies on animals before weaning are possible but require special techniques.[11,44] A species not closely related to rats and mice should also be tested in important cases to maximize the possibility of detecting behavioral toxicity.

## BROAD-SCALE DETECTION

Two general procedures are recommended for detecting behavioral toxicity, neither of which is unusually demanding in terms of special rooms, special skill in handling animals, or prolonged training of investigators. The first concerns the circadian rhythm of motor activity and ingestive behavior. The second examines operant behavior for changes produced by a substance. With both procedures, adequate repetition of experiments, the establishment of dose-response relationships, and concurrent controls are essential. Concurrent testing of agents with known effects (positive controls) aids in the interpretation of results.[19,26]

## CIRCADIAN CYCLE OF ACTIVITY

Many animals display clear-cut changes in activity patterns through the day. Prolonged measurement of activity over many daily cycles has long been used in biological studies.[32,34,37,38,39,43] The circadian cycle of activity is reproducible in laboratory animals. Changes in the pattern of this activity are a sensitive indicator of behavioral toxicity.[5,31,33]

Residential mazes have recently been employed to measure group activity of rats over relatively long periods.[32] Carefully placed photocells and light-emitting diodes record both amount and location of the activity of groups of four rats over several days. Cumulative hourly counts are usually recorded and nocturnal and diurnal activity separately examined. Food and water intake are also recorded. Behavioral hyper- or hypoactivity after exposure to toxic agents may be detected in this way. So also might short-term oscillations in activity, such as feeding-related cycles of rat activity during the nocturnal period, even though total circadian activity remains unaltered.[36] Published data demonstrate the ability of circadian measurements to detect effects of low doses of compounds that cause hyperactivity (e.g., amphetamine[31]), as well as effects of exposure to carbon monoxide,[5] X-irradiation,[33] or heavy metals such as inorganic lead.[36]

Other types of residential cages have been described,[2,7,38] but there is no evidence that cage design is a significant factor in the sensitivity of circadian activity to substances causing behavioral toxicity. Activity sensors, which can be added to any cage, record circadian activity of both large and small animals.

## OPERANT BEHAVIOR

Behavioral toxicity may also appear as altered performance of learned responses. Operant behavior is defined as behavior that is maintained by its own consequences. The operant behavior frequently studied in behavioral toxicology is maintained by precisely defined schedules of reinforcement. (Descriptions of the basic principles of operant behavior are readily available, with adequate accounts appearing in most undergraduate texts on experimental psychology.) Generally, with these procedures an animal works in an apparatus containing some sort of lever or key that closes a switch and a device to deliver reinforcers such as food or water. Operations of the switch are called responses. The circuitry is arranged so that occasional responses deliver the reinforcer. The response patterns depend on the schedule design, i.e., the precise way in which responses are allowed to produce the reinforcer. Various patterns of schedule-controlled response have proved sensitive and informative in drug studies. The extensive literature in behavioral pharmacology can now serve as the source of relevant techniques for the study of toxic substances.[14,15,21,48,49,53]

Behavioral toxicity in mice can be detected by a relatively simple and inexpensive method.[54] The mouse interrupts a beam of light to a photocell. This causes a dipper to deliver small quantities of milk according to a schedule. Two schedules that have been studied extensively are the fixed ratio (FR) and fixed interval (FI) schedules. Both may be used together so that data are collected on two distinct types of operant behavior during the same daily experimental session. For example, milk may be delivered alternately after 30 responses (an FR schedule) or at the first response after 300 s have elapsed FI schedule). Each schedule is associated with a distinctive external stimulus. Such schedules lead to characteristic patterns of response that are best displayed on a specially designed cumulative recorder. Evidence of behavioral toxicity is seen as both the pattern and the number of responses change.[10] There are a number of schedules used to study the toxic effects of chemicals.[1,9,27,29,52,53] There is also a very large amount of literature on their use in pharmacology.[28]

Preliminary training of the mice involves a partial food deprivation and a training sequence. Several sessions are needed, but, once trained, a mouse may be tested in daily sessions for a year or more. The performance remains consistent from day to day, permitting assessment of acute, subchronic, or chronic toxicity, as well as the degree and rate of the reversibility of effects.

Schedule-controlled responses can also be studied in other species. Monkeys, dogs, cats, rats, mice, pigeons, and others generally show similar patterns of response when the response is programmed to have consequences on a particular schedule.[6,22,23,51]

## CONFIRMATION OF IMPLICATIONS RESULTING FROM CHRONIC STUDIES

Behavioral or neurological effects suggested during other toxicological studies may be confirmed and quantified through further behavioral work. Because possible leads cannot be anticipated, the following examples are only illustrative. The detection of any behavioral deficit may well mean that other behavioral changes will be discovered, if appropriate techniques are applied.

Reported ataxia or weakness may be further studied by measuring the ability of a rat to remain on a rotating rod[24,50] or on a narrow, moving treadmill.[13] Tremors may be studied by putting rats on a displacement sensing device.[12,55] Hypo- or hyperreflexia shows as a decrease or increase in the auditory startle response.[16,20,41] In studies involving antenatal or neonatal exposure, toxicity may be manifested either as abnormal reflexes or as reflexes that appear at abnormal times in the animal's development.[11,40,45]

Operant conditioning procedures can be used to study specific behavioral functions. For example, it is possible to measure how well animals can space responses in time,[42] discriminate the amount of behavior just emitted,[25,35] or acquire complex behavior sequences.[3,47] One may anticipate the abuse potential of a substance by determining whether an animal will work for self-administration.[4] Suspected changes in visual, auditory, somesthetic, and proprioceptive sensory function may be assessed either by using reflex methods such as auditory startle (see above) or by training an animal to respond on the basis of particular sensory input. An introduction to much of this work has been provided by Stebbins[46] and Evans.[8] Many of these procedures can provide interesting and important detail on precise behavioral deficits. But they may be too technically difficult and expensive to be useful for the routine screening of toxic chemicals, despite the important role they play in basic research in behavioral toxicology. Therefore, only when information is needed about very important substances is the use of some of these techniques warranted. Further developmental work should produce methods that will soon allow us to test toxic agents more expeditiously.

## SUMMARY

Two general procedures have been recommended for use in the initial search for toxic behavioral effects of chemicals. One studies the circadian cycle of activity, the other operant behavior. They are believed to be sensitive, quantitatively reliable, and relatively easy to perform. These features are important where several doses of a compound, and perhaps several different groups of animals varying in age, sex, strain, or species, may be needed for an adequate evaluation. In addition, both procedures are suitable for the evaluation of the onset rate of an effect during exposure and the rate and completeness of recovery when exposure ceases, both extremely important features of behavioral toxicity.

Only relatively simple methods have been recommended for routine use. More elaborate and specific procedures should prove useful in elucidating the nature of any behavioral toxicity. Additional techniques, drawn from neurophysiology, neurocytology, and neurochemistry, would be required to explore fully the mechanisms of action of toxic chemicals. From a practical standpoint, the existence of behavioral toxicity at a particular exposure level is important in its own right, whatever the mechanisms of action. Behavioral toxicity may result from effects on a wide variety of organs and tissues. It is by no means an unequivocal indication of direct CNS toxicity.

Behavioral toxicology is still in an early stage of development, with systematic experimental studies appearing only recently.[17,18,19,52,53,56,57] No testing methods have been adequately validated through extensive use. A thorough reassessment of suggested procedures will be needed as more data become available.

## REFERENCES

1. Armstrong, R. D., L. J. Leach, P. R. Belluscio, E. A. Maynard, H. C. Hodge, and J. K. Scott. 1963. Behavioral changes in the pigeon following the inhalation of mercury vapor. Am. Ind. Hyg. Assoc. J. 24:366-375.
2. Barnett, S. A., and I. M. McEwan. 1973. Movements of virgin, pregnant and lactating mice in a residential maze. Physiol. Behav. 10:741-746.
3. Boren, J. J., and D. D. Devine. 1968. The repeated acquisition of behavioral chains. J. Exp. Anal. Behav. 11:651-660.
4. Cotten, M. deV., ed. 1975. Symposium on Control of Drug-Taking Behavior by Schedules of Reinforcement. Pharmacol. Rev. 27:287-548.
5. Culver, B., and S. Norton. 1976. Juvenile hyperactivity in rats after acute exposure to carbon monoxide. Exp. Neurol. 50:80-98.
6. Dews, P. B. 1958. Analysis of effects of psychopharmacological agents in behavioral terms. Fed. Proc. Fed. Am. Soc. Exp. Biol. 17:1024-1030.
7. Ely, D. L., E. G. Greene, and J. P. Henry. 1976. Minicomputer monitored social behavior of mice with hippocampus lesions. Behav. Biol. 16:1-29.
8. Evans, H. L. In press. Behavioral assessment in sensory toxicology. In: Zenick, H., and L. W. Reiter, eds. Behavioral Toxicology: An Emerging Discipline. Washington, D.C., Government Printing Office. Chapter 8.
9. Evans, H. L., V. G. Laties, and B. Weiss. 1975. Behavioral effects of mercury and methylmercury. Fed. Proc. Fed. Am. Soc. Exp. Biol. 34:1858-1867.
10. Ferster, C. B., and B. F. Skinner. 1957. Schedules of Reinforcement. New York, Appleton-Century-Crofts.
11. Fox, W. M. 1965. Reflex-ontogeny and behavioural development of the mouse. Anim. Behav. 13:234-241.
12. Frommel, E. 1965. The cholinergic mechanism of psychomotor agitation in apomorphine-injected mice. Arch. Int. Pharmacodyn. Ther. 154:231-234.
13. Gibbins, R. J., H. Kalant, and A. E. LeBlanc. 1968. A technique for accurate measurement of moderate degrees of alcohol intoxication in small animals. J. Pharmacol. Exp. Ther. 159:236-242.

14. Glick, S. D., and J. Goldfarb, eds. 1976. Behavioral Pharmacology. St. Louis, The C. V. Mosby Co.
15. Harvey, J. A., ed. 1971. Behavioral Analysis of Drug Action: Research and Commentary. Glenview, Ill., Scott, Foresman & Co.
16. Hoffman, H. S., and J. L. Searle. 1965. Acoustic variables in the modification of startle reaction in the rat. J. Comp. Physiol. Psychol. 60:53-58.
17. Horváth, M., ed. 1973. Adverse Effects of Environmental Chemicals and Psychotropic Drugs: Quantitative Interpretation of Functional Tests, vol. 1. Amsterdam, Elsevier.
18. Horváth, M., ed. 1976. Adverse Effects of Environmental Chemicals and Psychotropic Drugs: Neurophysiological and Behavioural Tests, vol. 2. Amsterdam, Elsevier.
19. Horváth, M., and E. Frantík. 1973. Quantitative interpretation of toxicological data: The use of reference substances. *In*: Horváth, M., ed. Adverse Effects of Environmental Chemicals and Psychotropic Drugs: Quantitative Interpretation of Functional Tests, vol. 1. Amsterdam, Elsevier. pp. 11-21.
20. Ison, J. R., and G. R. Hammond. 1971. Modification of the startle reflex in the rat by changes in the auditory and visual environments. J. Comp. Physiol. Psychol. 75:435-452.
21. Iversen, S. D., and L. L. Iversen. 1975. Behavioral Pharmacology. New York, Oxford University Press.
22. Kelleher, R. T., and W. H. Morse. 1968. Determinants of the specificity of behavioral effects of drugs. Ergeb. Physiol. Biol. Chem. Exp. Pharmakol. 60:1-56.
23. Kelleher, R. T., and W. H. Morse. 1968. Determinants of the behavioral effects of drugs. *In*: Tedeschi, D. H., and R. E. Tedeschi, eds. Importance of Fundamental Principles in Drug Evaluation. New York, Raven Press. pp. 383-405.
24. Kinnard, W. J., Jr., and C. J. Carr. 1957. A preliminary procedure for the evaluation of central nervous system depressants. J. Pharmacol. Exp. Ther. 121:354-361.
25. Laties, V. G. 1972. The modification of drug effects on behavior by external discriminative stimuli. J. Pharmacol. Exp. Ther. 183:1-13.
26. Laties, V. G. 1973. On the use of reference substances in behavioral toxicology. *In*: Horváth, M., ed. Adverse Effects of Environmental Chemicals and Psychotropic Drugs: Quantitative Interpretation of Functional Tests, vol. 1. Amsterdam, Elsevier. pp. 83-88.
27. Levine, T. E. 1976. Effects of carbon disulfide and FLA-63 on operant behavior in pigeons. J. Pharmacol. Exp. Ther. 199:669-678.
28. McMillan, D. E., and J. D. Leander. 1976. Effects of drugs on schedule-controlled behavior. *In*: Glick, S. D., and J. Goldfarb, eds. Behavioral Pharmacology. St. Louis, The C. V. Mosby Co. pp. 85-139.
29. McMillan, D. E., and A. T. Miller, Jr. 1974. Interactions between carbon monoxide and $d$-amphetamine or pentobarbital on schedule-controlled behavior. Environ. Res. 8:53-63.
30. National Academy of Sciences-National Research Council. 1975. Principles for Evaluating Chemicals in the Environment. Report prepared for the Environmental Protection Agency by the Environmental Studies Board and the Committee on Toxicology. Washington, D.C. Chapter 11, Effects on behavior, pp. 198-216.
31. Norton, S., B. Culver, and P. Mullenix. 1975. Measurement of the effects of drugs on activity of permanent groups of rats. Psychopharmacol. Commun. 1:131-138.
32. Norton, S., B. Culver, and P. Mullenix. 1975. Development of nocturnal behavior in albino rats. Behav. Biol. 15:317-331.
33. Norton, S., P. Mullenix, and B. Culver. 1976. Comparison of the structure of hyperactive behavior in rats after brain damage from X-irradiation, carbon monoxide and pallidal lesions. Brain Res. 116:49-67.
34. Pappenheimer, J. R., T. B. Miller, and C. A. Goodrich. 1967. Sleep-promoting effects of cerebrospinal fluid from sleep-deprived goats. Proc. Natl. Acad. Sci. USA 58:513-517.

35. Pliskoff, S. S., and I. Goldiamond. 1966. Some discriminative properties of fixed ratio performance in the pigeon. J. Exp. Anal. Behav. 9:1-9.
36. Reiter, L. W. In press. Observational techniques: Effects of lead on activity. *In*: Zenick, H., and L. W. Reiter, eds. Behavioral Toxicology: An Emerging Discipline. Washington, D.C., Government Printing Office. Chapter 6.
37. Richter, C. P. 1922. A behavioristic study of the activity of the rat. Comp. Psychol. Monogr. 1:1-55.
38. Ringle, D. A., and B. L. Herndon. 1969. Effect on rats of CSF from sleep-deprived rabbits. Pfleugers Arch. Gesamte Physiol. Menschen Tierre 306:320-328.
39. Robbins, T. W. 1977. A critique of the methods available for measurement of spontaneous motor activity. *In*: Iversen, L. L., and S. D. Iversen, eds. Handbook of Psychopharmacology, vol. 7. New York, Plenum. Chapter 2.
40. Rodier, P. M. In press. Postnatal functional evaluations. *In*: Wilson, J. G., and F. C. Fraser, eds. Handbook of Teratology, vol. 4. New York, Plenum.
41. Sagvolden, T., and K. Wester. 1974. Habituation of the startle reflex in rats with septal lesions. Behav. Biol. 12:413-418.
42. Sidman, M. 1955. Technique for assessing the effects of drugs on timing behavior. Science 122:925.
43. Slonaker, J. R. 1912. The normal activity of the albino rat from birth to natural death, its rate of growth and the duration of life. J. Anim. Behav. 2:20-42.
44. Spyker, J. M. 1975. Behavioral teratology and toxicology. *In*: Weiss, B., and V. G. Laties, eds. Behavioral Toxicology. New York, Plenum. pp. 311-349.
45. Spyker, J. M. 1975. Assessing the impact of low level chemicals on development: Behavioral and latent effects. Fed. Proc. Fed. Am. Soc. Exp. Biol. 34:1835-1844.
46. Stebbins, W. C., ed. 1970. Animal Psychophysics: The Design and Conduct of Sensory Experiments. New York, Appleton-Century-Crofts.
47. Thompson, D. M. 1973. Repeated acquisition as a behavioral base line for studying drug effects. J. Pharmacol. Exp. Ther. 184:506-514.
48. Thompson, T., and C. R. Schuster. 1968. Behavioral Pharmacology. Englewood Cliffs, N.J., Prentice-Hall, Inc.
49. Thompson, T., R. Pickens, and R. A. Meisch, eds. 1970. Readings in Behavioral Pharmacology. New York, Appleton-Century-Crofts.
50. Watzman, N., and H. Barry III. 1968. Drug effects on motor coordination. Psychopharmacologia 12:414-423.
51. Weiss, B., and V. G. Laties. 1967. Comparative pharmacology of drugs affecting behavior. Fed. Proc. Fed. Am. Soc. Exp. Biol. 26:1146-1156.
52. Weiss, B., and V. G. Laties, eds. 1975. Behavioral Toxicology. New York, Plenum.
53. Weiss, B., and V. G. Laties, eds. 1976. Behavioral Pharmacology: The Current Status. Originally appeared in Fed. Proc. Fed. Am. Soc. Exp. Biol., vol. 34, no. 9, Aug. 1975. First published in book form by Plenum, New York.
54. Wenger, G. R., and P. B. Dews. 1976. The effects of phencyclidine, ketamine, *d*-amphetamine and pentobarbital on schedule-controlled behavior in the mouse. J. Pharmacol. Exp. Ther. 196:616-624.
55. Word, T., and J. A. Stern. 1958. A simple stabilimeter. J. Exp. Anal. Behav. 1:201-203.
56. Xintaras, C., B. L. Johnson, and I. de Groot, eds. 1974. Behavioral Toxicology: Early Detection of Occupational Hazards. Washington, D.C., Government Printing Office. HEW Publication No. (NIOSH) 74-126.
57. Zenick, H., and L. W. Reiter, eds. In press. Behavioral Toxicology: An Emerging Discipline. Washington, D.C., Government Printing Office.

# Regulations under the Federal Hazardous Substances Act

Chapter II, Title 16
Code of Federal Regulations

## §1500.3  *Definitions*

(b)(4)(i)  "Hazardous substance" means: (A) Any substance or mixture of substances which is toxic, corrosive, an irritant, a strong sensitizer, flammable or combustible, or generates pressure through decomposition, heat, or other means, if such substance or mixture of substances may cause substantial personal injury or substantial illness during or as a proximate result of any customary or reasonable foreseeable handling or use, including reasonably foreseeable ingestion by children.

(5)  "Toxic" shall apply to any substance (other than a radioactive substance) which has the capacity to produce personal injury or illness to man through ingestion, inhalation, or absorption through any body surface.

(6)(i)  "Highly toxic" means any substance which falls within any of the following categories:

(A)  Produces death within 14 days in half or more than half of a group of 10 or more laboratory white rats each weighing between 200 and 300 grams, at a single dose of 50 milligrams or less per kilogram of body weight, when orally administered; or

(B)  Produces death within 14 days in half or more than half of a group of 10 or more laboratory white rats each weighing between 200 and 300 grams, when inhaled continuously for a period of 1 hour or less at an atmospheric concentration of 200 parts per million by volume or less of gas or vapor or 2 milligrams per liter by volume or less of mist or dust, provided such concentration is likely to be encountered by man when the substance is used in any reasonably foreseeable manner; or

119

(C) Produces death within 14 days in half or more than half of a group of 10 or more rabbits tested in a dosage of 200 milligrams or less per kilogram of body weight, when administered by continuous contact with the bare skin for 24 hours or less.

(ii) If the Commission finds that available data on human experience with any substance indicate results different from those obtained on animals in the dosages and concentrations specified in paragraph (b)(6)(i) of this section, the human data shall take precedence.

(7) "Corrosive" means any substance which in contact with living tissue will cause destruction of tissue by chemical action, but shall not refer to action on inanimate surfaces.

(8) "Irritant" means any substance not corrosive within the meaning of section 2(i) of the act [restated in paragraph (b)(7) of this section] which on immediate, prolonged, or repeated contact with normal living tissue will induce a local inflammatory reaction.

(9) "Strong sensitizer" means a substance which will cause on normal living tissue through an allergic or photodynamic process a hypersensitivity which becomes evident on reapplication of the same substance and which is designated as such by the Commission. Before designating any substance as a strong sensitizer, the Commission, upon consideration of the frequency of occurrence and severity of the reaction, shall find that the substance has a significant potential for causing hypersensitivity.

## §1500.41    *Method of testing toxic substances*

The method of testing the toxic substances referred to in §1500.3 (c)(1)-(ii)(C) and (2)(iii) is as follows:

(a) *Acute dermal toxicity (single exposure).*  In the acute exposures, the agent is held in contact with the skin by means of a sleeve for periods varying up to 24 hours. The sleeve, made of rubber dam or other impervious material, is so constructed that the ends are reinforced with additional strips and should fit snugly around the trunk of the animal. The ends of the sleeve are tucked, permitting the central portion to "balloon" and furnish a reservoir for the dose. The reservoir must have sufficient capacity to contain the dose without pressure. In the following table are given the dimensions of sleeves and the approximate body surface exposed to the test substance. The sleeves may vary in size to accommodate smaller or larger subjects. In the testing of unctuous materials that adhere readily to the skin, mesh wire screen may be employed instead of the sleeve. The screen is padded and raised approximately 2 centimeters from the exposed skin. In the case of dry powder preparations, the skin and substance are moistened with physiological saline prior to exposure. The sleeve or screen is then slipped over the gauze that holds the dose applied to the skin. In the case of finely divided powders, the measured dose is evenly distributed on cotton gauze which is then secured to the area of exposure.

Dimensions of Sleeves for Acute Dermal Toxicity Test (Test Animal Rabbits)

| Measurements in Centimeters | | Range of Weight of Animals (grams) | Average Area of Exposure $(cm^2)$ | Average Percentage of Total Body Surface |
|---|---|---|---|---|
| Diameter at Ends | Over-all Length | | | |
| 7.0 | 12.5 | 2,500-3,500 | 240 | 10.7 |

(b) *Preparation of test animals.* The animals are prepared by clipping the skin of the trunk free of hair. Approximately one-half of the animals are further prepared by making epidermal abrasions every 2 or 3 centimeters longitudinally over the area of exposure. The abrasions are sufficiently deep to penetrate the stratum corneum (horny layer of the epidermis) but not to disturb the derma; that is, not to obtain bleeding.

(c) *Procedures for testing.* The sleeve is slipped onto the animal which is then placed in a comfortable but immobilized position in a multiple animal holder. Selected doses of liquids and solutions are introduced under the sleeve. If there is slight leakage from the sleeve, which may occur during the first few hours of exposure, it is collected and reapplied. Dosage levels are adjusted in subsequent exposures (if necessary) to enable a calculation of a dose that would be fatal to 50 percent of the animals. This can be determined from mortality ratios obtained at various doses employed. At the end of 24 hours the sleeves or screens are removed, the volume of unabsorbed material (if any) is measured, and the skin reactions are noted. The subjects are cleaned by thorough wiping, observed for gross symptoms of poisoning, and then observed for 2 weeks.

§1500.41   *Methods of testing primary irritant substances*

Primary irritation to the skin is measured by a patch-test technique on the abraded and intact skin of the albino rabbit, clipped free of hair. A minimum of six subjects are used in abraded and intact skin tests. Introduce under a square patch, such as surgical gauze measuring 1 inch by 1 inch and two single layers thick, 0.5 milliliter (in the case of liquids) or 0.5 grams (in the case of solids and semisolids) of the test substance. Dissolve solids in an appropriate solvent and apply the solution as for liquids. The animals are immobilized with patches secured in place by adhesive tape. The entire trunk of the animal is then wrapped with an impervious material, such as rubberized cloth, for the 24-hour period of exposure. This material aids in maintaining the test patches in position and retards the evaporation of volatile substances. After 24 hours of exposure, the patches are removed and the resulting reactions are evaluated on the basis of the designated values in the following table:

| Skin Reaction | Value[1] |
| --- | --- |
| Erythema and eschar formation: | |
| No erythema | 0 |
| Very slight erythema (barely perceptible) | 1 |
| Well-defined erythema | 2 |
| Moderate to severe erythema | 3 |
| Severe erythema (beet redness) to slight eschar formation (injuries in depth) | 4 |
| Edema formation: | |
| No edema | 0 |
| Very slight edema (barely perceptible) | 1 |
| Slight edema (edges of area well defined by definite raising) | 2 |
| Moderate edema (raised approximately 1 millimeter) | 3 |
| Severe edema (raised more than 1 millimeter and extending beyond | |
| the area of exposure) | 4 |

[1] The "value" recorded for each reading is the average value of the six or more animals subject to the test.

Readings are again made at the end of a total of 72 hours (48 hours after the first reading). An equal number of exposures are made on areas of skin that have been previously abraded. The abrasions are minor incisions through the stratum corneum, but not sufficiently deep to disturb the derma or to produce bleeding. Evaluate the reactions of the abraded skin at 24 hours and 72 hours, as described in this paragraph. Add the values for erythema and eschar formation at 24 hours and at 72 hours for intact skin to the values on abraded skin at 24 hours and at 72 hours (four values). Similarly, add the values for edema formation at 24 hours and at 72 hours for intact and abraded skin (four values). The total of the eight values is divided by four to give the primary irritation score. Example:

| Skin Reaction | Exposure Time (hours) | Exposure Unit (value) |
| --- | --- | --- |
| Erythema and eschar formation: | | |
| Intact skin | 24 | 2 |
| Do | 72 | 1 |
| Abraded skin | 24 | 3 |
| Do | 72 | 2 |
| Subtotal | | 8 |
| Edema formation: | | |
| Intact skin | 24 | 0 |
| Do | 72 | 1 |
| Abraded skin | 24 | 1 |
| Do | 72 | 2 |
| Subtotal | | 4 |
| Total | | 12 |

Thus, the primary irritation score is $12 \div 4 = 3$.

## §1500.42   *Test for eye irritants*

(a)(1)  Six albino rabbits are used for each test.substance. Animal facilities for such procedures shall be so designed and maintained as to exclude sawdust, wood chips, or other extraneous materials that might produce eye irritation. Both eyes of each animal in the test groups shall be examined before testing, and only those animals without eye defects or irritation shall be used. The animal is held firmly but gently until quiet. The test material is placed in one eye of each animal by gently pulling the lower lid away from the eyeball to form a cup into which the test substance is dropped. The lids are then gently held together for one second and the animal is released. The other eye, remaining untreated, serves as a control. For testing liquids, 0.1 milliliter is used. For solids or pastes, 100 milligrams of the test substance is used, except that for substances in flake, granule, powder, or other particulate form the amount that has a volume of 0.1 milliliter (after compacting as much as possible without crushing or altering the individual particles, such as by tapping the measuring container) shall be used whenever this volume weighs less than 100 milligrams. In such a case, the weight of the 0.1 milliliter test dose should be recorded. The eyes are not washed following instillation of test material except as noted below.

(2)  The eyes are examined and the grade of ocular reaction is recorded at 24, 48, and 72 hours. Reading of reactions is facilitated by use of a binocular loupe, hand slit-lamp, or other expert means. After the recording of observations at 24 hours, any or all eyes may be further examined after applying fluorescein. For this optional test, one drop of fluorescein sodium ophthalmic solution U.S.P. or equivalent is dropped directly on the cornea. After flushing out the excess fluorescein with sodium chloride solution U.S.P. or equivalent, injured areas of the cornea appear yellow: this is best visualized in a darkened room under ultraviolet illumination. Any or all eyes may be washed with sodium chloride solution U.S.P. or equivalent after the 24-hour reading.

(b)(1)  An animal shall be considered as exhibiting a positive reaction if the test substance produces at any of the readings ulceration of the cornea (other than a fine stippling), or opacity of the cornea (other than a slight dulling of the normal luster), or inflammation of the iris (other than a slight deepening of the folds (or rugae) or a slight circumcorneal injection of the blood vessels), or if such substance produces in the conjunctivae (excluding the cornea and iris) an obvious swelling with partial eversion of the lids or a diffuse crimson-red with individual vessels not easily discernible.

(2)  The test shall be considered positive if four or more of the animals in the test group exhibit a positive reaction. If only one animal exhibits a positive reaction, the test shall be regarded as negative. If two or three animals exhibit a positive reaction, the test is repeated using a different group of six animals.

The second test shall be considered positive if three or more of the animals exhibit a positive reaction. If only one or two animals in the second test exhibit a positive reaction, the test shall be repeated with a different group of six animals. Should a third test be needed, the substance will be regarded as an irritant if any animal exhibits a positive response.

(c) To assist testing laboratories and other interested persons in interpreting the results obtained when a substance is tested in accordance with the method described in paragraph (a) of this section, an "Illustrated Guide for Grading Eye Irritation by Hazardous Substances" will be sold by the Superintendent of Documents, U.S. Government Printing Office, Washington, D.C. 20402. The guide will contain color plates depicting responses of varying intensity to specific test solutions. The grade of response and the substance used to produce the response will be indicated.

(38 FR 27012, Sept. 27, 1973; 38 FR 30105, Nov. 1, 1973)

REPRINTED FROM FEDERAL REGISTER, 41 (188): 42501
SEPTEMBER 27, 1976

§173.240  *Corrosive material; definition.*

(a) For the purpose of this subchapter, a corrosive material is a liquid or solid that causes visible destruction or irreversible alterations in human skin tissue at the site of contact, or in the case of leakage from its packaging, a liquid that has a severe corrosion rate on steel.

(1) A material is considered to be destructive or to cause irreversible alteration in human skin tissue if when tested on the intact skin of the albino rabbit by the technique described in Appendix A to this part, the structure of the tissue at the site of contact is destroyed or changed irreversibly after an exposure period of 4 hours or less.

(2) A liquid is considered to have a severe corrosion rate if its corrosion rate exceeds 0.250 inch per year (IPY) on steel (SAE 1020) at a test temperature of 130°F. An acceptable test is described in NACE Standard TM-01-69.

(b) If human experience or other data indicate that the hazard of a material is greater or less than indicated by the results of the tests specified in paragraph (a) of this section, the Department may revise its classification or make the material subject to the requirements of Parts 170-189 of this subchapter.

[Amdt. 173-61, 37 FR 5947, Mar. 23, 1972; as amended by Amdt. 173-74, 38 FR 20839, Aug. 3, 1973; Amdt. 173-94, 41 FR 16074, Apr. 15, 1976]

# Animal
# B Husbandry

*Animal quality.* It serves no useful purpose either to purchase a low-quality microbially undefined animal for a high-security barrier operation or to place germfree animals in conventional, nonbarrier facilities. The nature and risks of the experiment dictate the quality of the animal and environmental controls. Purchased animals must be properly transported and quarantined upon arrival to assure continued high quality.

Operational and extraneous factors can have dramatic effects on the successful completion of a chronic test, as well as on the interpretation and usefulness of the results. Contaminants in the diet, bedding, water, or air can introduce variables or modifiers to chronic toxicity. Other factors, such as intercurrent infections, autolysis, and cannibalism, can reduce the effective number of animals in the study; however, these are largely preventable by the routine practice of strict hygiene-disease prevention measures and close clinical observation.

*Facilities.* Good physical design and maintenance of the animal facilities are required in order to meet the high standards of animal care, and the chemical and biological hazard control required for chronic toxicity studies. Even the best animals placed in poorly designed and maintained facilities will soon succumb to their surroundings.

The construction or modification of animal facilities to be used for long-term studies should provide practical but effective barriers to the inadvertent introduction of infectious diseases or contaminants into the facility or between animal rooms. As a minimum, the design should include a unidirectional flow

125

of equipment, supplies, air, and personnel. This is usually referred to as the "clean-dirty (return) corridor" concept. The doors to animal rooms should be located at opposite ends of each room. All materials are sterilized; personnel are fully covered in sterilized garments; and entrances are restricted to clean corridor and exits to the dirty corridor. Such a strict flow of materials and personnel through a corridor from which access to other rooms is impossible greatly reduces the potential for introduction of disease to the facility or the rapid spread of a disease from one room to part or all of the facility. Where such a corridor arrangement is not possible, the movement of clean and dirty equipment and materials should be scheduled to avoid back-flow to cleaner areas. Animal rooms must be protected to reduce possible contamination between rooms.

A committee of the National Academy of Sciences[1] has recently established a new classification for barrier systems based on methods and extent of contamination control. Classification consists of maximum, high, moderate, or minimal security and conventional systems. Minimal security conventional systems are not considered acceptable for maintaining rodents for long periods.

The animal facilities should be separated from the remainder of the laboratories with access restricted to essential personnel. A special quarantine area, effectively separated from the testing area, should be provided for holding animals procured from outside the animal facility.

Small rooms are recommended for chronic toxicity testing so that a separate room can be used for each species and test agent. This allows for better prevention and easier containment of a disease outbreak. It also prevents inadvertent exposure of animals to low levels of other chemicals, which could result if several chemicals were on test in the same room. This arrangement also reduces the possibility of accidental mixup in the test groups of treatment administrations and the introduction of diseased animals into a room in which studies are under way. The increased cost incurred by using these small rooms is considered a warranted expense. When large rooms must be used, a reasonable compromise is the use of cages with solid sides and bottoms and covered by filter tops.

All air entering and leaving the animal facilities should be adequately filtered with 10 to 15 fresh-air changes per hour. Provisions for the automatic control and recording of temperature and humidity in each room should be provided along with a monitoring system to alert the attendants to any deviations from the acceptable range.

*Equipment/Supplies.* To complement an adequately designed facility, equipment and supplies should be of suitable construction or composition and capable of effective sanitization.

Numerous studies have been lost due to unforeseen failures in mechanical equipment (especially the air-conditioning system) or to food supply problems caused by labor disputes, mill shortages, etc. Rotated, reserve backup supplies should be maintained to ensure continued food supplies. Air-conditioning failures can be due to such malfunctions as compressor failure or interruption of electricity. Access to an emergency generator or parallel air-conditioning system should be an integral part of any facility contingency plan.

Several commercially available rack/caging systems are capable of proper sanitization. Plastic or stainless steel cages with solid sides and bottoms covered with nonwoven polyester fiber filters constitute an effective enclosure and provide for relatively efficient disease control and chemical containment measures. However, the gains from the additional environmental control may be partially offset by elevated cage humidity and ammonia levels, which might have the detrimental effects of respiratory disorders and hepatic enzyme induction. Wire mesh cages may be required for certain studies such as those of inhalation. During the quarantine period and short-term toxicity studies, animals may be caged together according to weight-space specifications recommended by the National Academy of Sciences. However, for the sub-chronic and chronic studies, animals should be distributed from the outset of the studies as if they were in the upper weight range. This will obviate the need for later redistribution to keep them within the weight-space specifications.

Although mycotoxin-free ground corncob may be used for bedding, heat-treated hardwood chips are more desirable. Softwood chips or creosoted wood should not be used. The bedding should be sterilized. When open wire mesh cages are used, an absorbent material should be placed under the cages to collect and hold waste matter.

Feeders designed to prevent soiling, bridging, and scattering of the feed are acceptable when pellet-type rations are used. Although no feeder is completely satisfactory for meal feed, a hopper-type feeder that is firmly attached to the cage appears to cause the fewest problems. However, this type of feeder may still require daily "bumping" to dislodge bridged meal. An open, unfixed feed cup should not be used, nor should the feed be placed directly onto the cage floor.

Water systems should provide an adequate continuous supply of fresh, pathogen-free water. When an automatic watering system is used, the valve end should be positioned so that accidental flooding of the cage is avoided.

*Operations.* The key to a successful animal care operation is a well-trained and motivated caretaker staff interested in and concerned with the health of the individual animals and their role in quality research. As in design considerations, operations should strive to prevent entrance of extraneous factors at all levels of containment, from facility to animal room to individual cage.

Lack of or improper quarantine with inadvertent introduction of disease to a facility can jeopardize chronic studies that may have been under way for many months. Strict procedures in this regard are essential. Newly arrived animals should be taken, in their unopened shipping containers, directly to the quarantine area. Those unsuitable because of size, health, or other criteria should be immediately discarded; remaining animals should be quarantined and closely monitored for a minimum of 7 days. A small, randomly selected number of animals from each shipment should be sacrificed and examined for parasites and enteric pathogens. When an epizootic disease is found among the animals, the entire shipment from which they came should be discarded. Professional judgment must be exercised to determine whether minor losses should be attributed to the stress of shipment or to normal attrition of young animals.

Access to the animal facilities should be restricted to essential personnel. Both professional and technical personnel should receive training in animal care and personal hygiene. Those with disease conditions that could affect the animals' health should not be permitted in the animal rooms.

Attention should also be given to supplies entering the facility or animal rooms to prevent introduction of disease. The measures used should conform to the disease prevention plan, e.g., barrier or conventional operation, etc. The sterilizing of food and bedding, as well as the showering of personnel, while warranted in barrier and clean/dirty corridor facilities, may not be practical for many conventional operations.

Early detection of impending problems, as well as the documentation of perturbations that might be used in data interpretation, can be accomplished by monitoring the environment. The physical environment (temperature, humidity, airflow, etc.), should be monitored for deviations from acceptable range, while supplies (food, bedding, and water) should be monitored for proper composition and presence of biological and chemical contaminants. Animals and their discharges can be monitored for microorganisms and parasites.

Whenever individual animal data are to be routinely recorded, each animal should be marked at the outset of the study with a standard method of identification, such as ear notching, toe clipping, or tagging.

## REFERENCE

1. National Academy of Sciences-National Research Council, Institute of Laboratory Animal Resources. 1972. Guide for the Care and Use of Laboratory Animals, rev. ed. Washington, D.C., Government Printing Office. DHEW Publication No. (NIH) 74-23.

# C Hematological and Clinical Biochemistry Studies

Suggested list of tests for monitoring toxic effects and the health status of animals:

| Hematology | Clinical Chemistry |
|---|---|
| Total erythocyte counts | Blood urea nitrogen |
| Total leukocyte counts | SGPT |
| Hematocrit | SGOT |
| Hemoglobin | Alkaline phosphatase |
| Differential leukocyte counts | |

# D  Pathology

Suggested list of organs used to obtain relative organ weights:

| Brain | Heart | Adrenals |
| Lungs | Kidneys | Gonads |
| Liver | Spleen | |

Suggested list of tissues for histopathology:

| Brain | Pituitary | Salivary gland |
| Thyroids | Trachea | Peribronchial lymph node |
| Heart | Lung (*in toto*) | Liver |
| Kidneys | Spleen | Stomach |
| Small intestine | Pancreas | Mesenteric lymph node |
| Large intestine | Gonads | Bone marrow |
| Bone | Prostate | Skeletal muscle |
| Peripheral nerve | Eye | Uterus |
| Skin | Nasal cavity | Gross abnormalities |
| | | Urinary bladder |